T0133435

The Changing Roles of Doctors

Edited by

PENELOPE CAVENAGH

PhD, MSc, BSc, DMS, Dip CSLT, C Psychol
*Director of Research and Enterprise and
Head of The Graduate School, University Campus Suffolk*

SAM J LEINSTER

BSc, MD, FRCS (Edin & Eng), SFHEA, FAcadMEd
*Emeritus Professor of Medical Education and
former Dean, Norwich Medical School, University of East Anglia*

SUSAN MILES

BA(Hons), PhD, MBPsS, CSci
*Research Associate in Medical Education
Norwich Medical School, University of East Anglia*

Foreword by
SIR KENNETH CALMAN

Radcliffe Publishing
London • New York

Radcliffe Publishing Ltd
33–41 Dallington Street
London
EC1V 0BB
United Kingdom
www.radcliffehealth.com

British Library Cataloguing in Publication Data

A catalogue record for this book is available from the British Library.

ISBN-13: 978 184619 991 2

The paper used for the text pages of this book
is FSC® certified. FSC (The Forest Stewardship
Council®) is an international network to promote
responsible management of the world's forests.

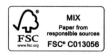

Typeset by Darkriver Design, Auckland, New Zealand
Printed and bound by TJI Digital, Padstow, Cornwall

Contents

Foreword

All professional groups are subject to change over time, but the last few decades have seen an acceleration in this change. There are many reasons for this, including the rise of associated professional groups, changes in the demography of the client base, and the clients' greater knowledge base and understanding of the issues. All of these aspects of change are positive, but the professional group does not always interpret them in that way. Doctors are not an exception to such changes, so how should they respond, and how should they continue to serve patients with the same values and professional ethos? This book begins to tackle and analyse such issues by discussing a range of matters that are relevant to the management of change. The profession of medicine, viewed from the outside, is often seen as conservative, and numerous examples over the years have shown opportunities that have been missed or delayed. The profession sometimes seems to react to events rather than leading and creating opportunities, so with the pace of change increasing now is a good time to consider things in depth.

It is perhaps worth first considering the role of the doctor, before discussing the factors that influence change and which need to be considered in looking to the future. What are doctors for, and is the purpose something that is long-lasting, or does it change with time? This consideration may or may not be irrespective of the setting, the knowledge of the patients, and the size and shape of the clinical team.

So what do doctors do? What are their boundaries with other professional groups, and how should they relate and interact with patients and the public? In a book written a few years ago, I suggested that the aim of medicine might be as follows.

> The aim of medicine is to assist in the process of healing in its broadest sense – both of individuals and of communities . . . Doctors do this by improving quality of life, providing care, relieving suffering, promoting health and preventing illness and disease. This aim is grounded in the understanding of health and the

mechanisms of illness and disease, which then forms the basis of effective and appropriate treatment. Doctors must do this in full cooperation with the patient, public and other providers of health care. (KC Calman, *Medical Education: past, present and future.* Churchill Livingstone, 2007, page 347)

This might seem rather lofty and divorced from reality, but most of the topics in this book touch on this definition one way or another, whether it is related to the changing work environment, educational initiatives, revalidation, or working as part of a team. The governance of this is critical if the profession is to serve the public – hence issues of management regulation and the measurement of outcome.

The profession of medicine is changing, more rapidly perhaps than many doctors think. Whether it relates to the professional power base or the changing demographics of the profession itself, both topics are discussed in this book. The topics are thought-provoking, as they should be, but all come back to asking what doctors are for. This remains a key issue and one that requires discussion and debate.

Sir Kenneth Calman
February 2013

About the editors

Dr Penelope Cavenagh, PhD, MSc, BSc, DMS, Dip CSLT, C Psychol
**Director of Research and Enterprise and Head of The Graduate
School at University Campus Suffolk**

Dr Cavanagh is Visiting Professor at the University of East Anglia
and an honorary Professor at Essex University. She is an experienced
health service researcher and has published extensively in the area
of doctors moving into management roles. Her PhD is in the area
of medical management and medical education. She is a chartered
psychologist and has also been a non-executive Director of an
Acute Hospital Foundation Trust for 11 years. She is also one of the
co-editors and authors of *The Changing Face of Medical Education*
(Radcliffe Publishing, 2011).
   Email: p.cavenagh@ucs.ac.uk

Professor Sam J Leinster, BSc, MD, FRCS (Edin & Eng), SFHEA, FAcadMEd
**Emeritus Professor of Medical Education and former Dean,
Norwich Medical School, University of East Anglia**

Professor Leinster has been a leading breast surgeon who helped to
found the University of East Anglia's innovative undergraduate medical curriculum. He was previously Director of Medical Studies and
Professor of Surgery at the University of Liverpool, where he established the Breast Unit – one of the leaders in the United Kingdom
– at The Royal Liverpool Hospital. He is involved nationally in
many aspects of medical education and is also one of the co-editors
and authors of *The Changing Face of Medical Education* (Radcliffe
Publishing, 2011).
   Email: S.Leinster@uea.ac.uk

Dr Susan Miles, BA(Hons), PhD, MBPsS, CSci
**Research Associate in Medical Education, Norwich Medical School,
University of East Anglia**

Dr Miles is a research psychologist and chartered scientist who actively researches and publishes in medical education. She is also one of the co-editors and authors of *The Changing Face of Medical Education* (Radcliffe Publishing, 2011).

Email: susan.miles@uea.ac.uk

List of contributors

Professor Ann Barrett, OBE, MD, FRCR, FRCP, is Emeritus Professor of Oncology at the University of East Anglia (UEA) and was formerly Deputy Dean of the Norwich Medical School, UEA, and lead clinician for oncology at the Norfolk and Norwich University Hospital NHS Trust.
Email: a.barrett@doctors.org.uk

Dr Ian LP Beales, BSc (Hons), MB BS (Hons), MD, FRCP (London), FHEA, FEBG, MAcadMEd, is Clinical Senior Lecturer in Cell Biology and Gastroenterology at the University of East Anglia and Honorary Consultant Gastroenterologist at the Norfolk and Norwich University Hospital. He is also the Training Programme Director and Head of Specialty Training for the East of England Gastroenterology Training scheme, and Co-Director of the Norwich Endoscopy Training Centre.
Email: I.Beales@uea.ac.uk

Dr Laura Bowater, BSc (Hons), MSc, MAHEP, PhD, is a Senior Lecturer in Medical Education at the Norwich Medical School, University of East Anglia.
Email: Laura.Bowater@uea.ac.uk

Dr Bernard Thomas Brett, BSc, MB BS, FRCP (Lon), AMM (BAMM), is currently the Deputy Medical Director and Responsible Officer at the James Paget University Hospitals NHS Foundation Trust (JPUH) and was formerly the Medical Director from 2009 to 2012. He is also a Consultant Gastroenterologist and a Consultant Physician at the JPUH.
Email: bernard.brett@jpaget.nhs.uk

Dr Mick Collins, PhD, BSc (Hons), Dip HSc, Cert Ed, is a Lecturer in Occupational Therapy in the Faculty of Medicine and Health Sciences at the University of East Anglia.
Email: Mick.Collins@uea.ac.uk

Dr Sandra Gibson, BSc (Hons), PhD, PGCE, FHEA, is a Senior Lecturer in Medical Education and Head of Assessment and Information at the Norwich Medical School, University of East Anglia.

    Email: S.Gibson@uea.ac.uk

Professor Christopher H Hand, MA, MSc, MB BChir, FRCP, FRCGP, is a retired general practitioner in Bungay, Suffolk. Until his recent retirement he was a Deputy Course Director of the Bachelor of Medicine and Bachelor of Surgery programme at the Norwich Medical School, University of East Anglia.

    Email: drchand@gotadsl.co.uk

Professor Amanda Howe, MA, MD, FRCGP, FAcadMEd, is a Clinical Professor of Primary Care at the Norwich Medical School, University of East Anglia. She is also an academic general practitioner at Bowthorpe Surgery in Norwich.

    Email: Amanda.Howe@uea.ac.uk

Joanne Kellett, BA Hons, is a Research Associate at the Norfolk and Norwich University Hospitals NHS Foundation Trust.

    Email: Joanne.Kellett@nnuh.nhs.uk

Alistair Leinster, BSc, PG Cert, MBA, is a General Manager working within the Alder Hey Children's NHS Foundation Trust.

    Email: aleinster@gmail.com

Dr Susanne Lindqvist, BSc, MSc, PhD, QTS, is a Lecturer in Interprofessional Practice in the Centre for Interprofessional Practice, Faculty of Medicine and Health Sciences at the University of East Anglia.

    Email: S.Lindqvist@uea.ac.uk

Dr Veena Rodrigues, MBBS, MD, MPhil, MClinEd, FFPH, is a Clinical Senior Lecturer in Public Health at the Norwich Medical School, University of East Anglia, and an honorary Consultant in Public Health Medicine, NHS Norfolk and Waveney.

    Email: V.Rodrigues@uea.ac.uk

Professor Krishna Sethia, DM, FRCS, is a Consultant Urologist and Medical Director of the Norfolk and Norwich University Hospitals NHS Foundation Trust.

    Email: krishna.sethia@nnuh.nhs.uk

Dr Andrea Stöckl, MA, MSc, PhD, is a Medical Anthropologist and Lecturer in Medical Sociology at the Norwich Medical School, University of East Anglia.

Email: A.Stockl@uea.ac.uk

Dr Richard Young, MA, MB BChir, FRCGP, DRCOG, FHEA, is an honorary Senior Lecturer and Lead Practice Development Tutor at the Norwich Medical School, University of East Anglia.

Email: D.Young@uea.ac.uk

CHAPTER 1

Drivers for change in the medical profession

Sam J Leinster

INTRODUCTION

The medical profession is an ancient and increasingly diverse institution. Both its status and its role in society have varied with time and place, but the pace of change has accelerated in the past 100 years. This chapter will attempt to survey these changes with particular reference to the United Kingdom. The effects of legislation and the structure of healthcare delivery will differ from country to country. The effects of developments in medical science and changes in professional attitudes will be more widely applicable.

FROM CARE TO CURE

The image of the ideal doctor is constantly changing. One of the most evocative pictures of the nineteenth-century image of the doctor is the painting by Sir Luke Fildes entitled simply *The Doctor*, first exhibited in 1891 but drawing on the experience of the death of his first son at the age of 1 year in 1877.[1] The doctor in this painting is clearly caring, concerned and thoughtful, but there is a strong impression that he has little to offer in the way of effective intervention. Interestingly, although the artist is drawing on his own experience, he has chosen to make the setting of the painting the home of a poor family, implying an expectation that the doctor would provide this care for patients based on need rather than their ability to pay.

As the twentieth century progressed, the effective interventions available to the doctor increased exponentially. The discovery of antibiotic agents in the 1930s and 1940s gave doctors the ability to treat life-threatening infections. By the 1960s there was a widespread belief that infective illnesses were no longer a major threat, provided medical treatment was available. The issue became a sociopolitical one of how the benefits of modern medicine could be accessed by the whole world population. The advent of anaesthesia, asepsis and biomedical engineering led to rapid developments in surgery including neurosurgery, cardiac surgery and organ transplantation. New imaging modalities and new laboratory techniques led to major improvements in diagnosis. The image of the ideal doctor shifted from that of caregiver to that of deliverer of cure. The measure of effective healthcare is not how the patient felt about the experience but, rather, what clinical outcomes were achieved.[2] The implicit model was that the body is a machine and the doctor is a technician with the knowledge and skills needed to maintain the machine and repair it if it goes wrong. Within this model, the depth and extent of the doctor's knowledge is more important than his or her ability to relate to the patient.

The increase in breadth and depth of knowledge has resulted in increasing specialisation and sub-specialisation as medical science developed. In the nineteenth century it was still possible for the well-educated physician to have a sound knowledge of the whole of medical practice and its underpinning scientific foundations. By the end of the twentieth century, knowledge was expanding so rapidly that one could only keep up to date by focusing on a relatively narrow spectrum of practice. In the author's own specialty of breast cancer, the Web of Knowledge research platform lists more than 48 428 papers in 2011 alone. Information that is important for improving the management of patients can get lost in the sheer volume of material.

The downside of sub-specialisation is that no one is in a position to take an overview of the patient's condition. The success of modern medicine in prolonging life expectancy has meant that chronic conditions have replaced acute illness as the main focus of medical care. Patients rarely present with a single pathology and are often under the care of several different specialists, each one of who has only a limited understanding of the conditions for which he or she is not directly responsible. Treatments that are effective for one condition may be detrimental for another from which the patient suffers. Added to this, many modern therapies are associated with side effects so that improvement in one condition may result in an overall deterioration in the health status of the patient. Fragmentation of care is often associated with neglect of the patient's psychosocial well-being.[3] This in turn may lead to poorer clinical outcomes.

An increasing awareness of the problems associated with a focus on the condition rather than the person has led to a swing back to a more holistic approach to medicine and a resurgence in the status of the general practitioner (GP), often known now as the primary care physician or the family physician. Paradoxically, general practice has become a specialty in its own right, with a growing emphasis on the management of patients with chronic conditions within a community setting.[4] Care has returned to the agenda.

FROM INDEPENDENT GUILD TO REGULATED PROFESSION

The accepted roles of the medical profession and its relationship to the rest of society have been defined in the past in a variety of codes, the best known of which, in the Western world, is the Hippocratic oath. The earliest code is, probably, the Oath of the Hindu Physicians, dating from the fifteenth century BC, while the most recent to gain widespread acceptance is the Declaration of Geneva, which was first produced by the World Medical Association in 1948 and was most recently revised in 2006. There is remarkable agreement between the codes on the roles and responsibilities of a physician, but there is no common mechanism for ensuring that practitioners adhere to the requirements of the codes.[5]

Medical practice in the United Kingdom in the first half of the nineteenth century was in the hands of a range of different professions of varying status within the community. The most highly regarded were the physicians, who were usually university trained and who were regulated by the College of Physicians in London if they practised in England, or by the College of Physicians of Edinburgh, Glasgow or Dublin if they practised in one of those cities. Their services were expensive and were, therefore, largely limited to the wealthy. Apothecaries, who acted as a cross between a GP and a pharmacist, served the general population. They compounded and dispensed drugs from neighbourhood shops but they also made diagnoses and prescribed treatment. Their training was apprenticeship based and they were regulated by the Society of Apothecaries. A third regulated profession was the surgeons. In addition to carrying out the limited range of surgery that was possible before the development of anaesthesia and antisepsis, they provided general medical care alongside the apothecaries. There was friction between the two professions, with complaints being made that the surgeons were working beyond their training and competence,[6] but it was not uncommon for individual practitioners to have dual training. In addition to the regulated practitioners, there were a large number of other people offering cures of varying description. Some of these were traditional healers making use of remedies and techniques handed down in families; others were charlatans deliberately exploiting the need and gullibility of the ill.

In response to growing public concern about the standards of medical practice, the UK government in 1858 established the General Council for Medical Education and Registration, later to be called the General Medical Council (GMC), whose functions were to define the minimum standards for training as a doctor and to maintain a register of those practitioners who had satisfied those standards.[7] The original council was drawn from members of the medical profession, elected by their peers, and supplemented by members nominated by major medical institutions, including those universities with a medical school. Although responsible to Parliament, the Council was seen by the profession and the public as a self-regulatory body for the medical profession. Removal from the register would only occur if the doctor were found to be guilty of serious professional misconduct. If a complaint was made against a doctor, the Professional Misconduct Committee of the GMC was responsible for investigating the complaint, prosecuting the doctor if deemed necessary, and making a judgement on the case. Lesser sanctions included the issue of a reprimand or suspension from the register for a fixed period.

Individuals who were not on the register could still practise medicine, but they could not advertise themselves as registered practitioners. They were restricted in their scope of practice and were not entitled to sign statutory certificates or work for government bodies, including (when it was established in 1948) the National Health Service (NHS).

A series of serious incidents in the 1990s, culminating in the case of Dr Harold Shipman, who was convicted of serial killings, led to the government setting up an independent review under the chairmanship of Dame Janet Smith, a High Court judge.[8] Following the recommendations from the inquiry major reforms of the GMC took place. The current council is appointed rather than elected and 50% of the membership is non-medical. In addition to being registered, a doctor now needs to be licensed in order to practise. Licensure requires renewal at 5-year intervals and is to be linked to revalidation, with each doctor being required to demonstrate that he or she has kept up to date in knowledge and skills and that he or she remains in good standing with professional colleagues[9] (*see* Chapter 8).

FROM HAPHAZARD TRAINING TO UNIFORM EDUCATION

Gradually, the training for aspiring doctors became more uniform, and by the end of the nineteenth century all entrants to the medical profession in the United Kingdom attended a recognised medical school. In London the schools were closely related to the major teaching hospitals. In Scotland and the English provinces they were usually part of the local university. In both systems the curriculum comprised a preclinical component of basic biological science followed by a period of clinical education on the hospital wards. This approach was strengthened by the publication in the United States of the Flexner Report in 1910,[10] which recommended that medical education should combine a strong scientific education with experiential clinical training at the patient's bedside.

The Education Committee of the GMC from the beginning set out standards for the education of doctors. Initially, the recommendations were couched in broad terms, defining the disciplines with which the newly qualified doctor should be familiar, rather than specifying details of the expected skills and knowledge. The doctor who qualified under this system was expected to be able to provide an acceptable standard of care across the whole range of medical disciplines, from internal medicine to obstetrics and surgery. However, specialisation was already a reality and some of the graduates chose to do further training within the teaching hospital setting in order, in due course, to practise as a specialist within a hospital. In many cases they were required to pay the hospital authorities for the privilege of working in the hospital during their period of training. Once they had reached a satisfactory level of training (not formally defined), they could apply for a post on the consultant staff of the hospital. In the more prestigious hospitals this appointment did not carry any remuneration; the consultant still ran an independent practice but was more likely to attract patients because of the hospital connection, which acted as a guarantee to the patient of the doctor's abilities.

Those who chose not to undergo further training could set up as GPs. A number of options were open to them. They could just open a practice in a given area and hope that patients would come to them in sufficient numbers to provide them with a livelihood. They could buy an established practice from a doctor who was retiring, or they could become an assistant to a successful GP, perhaps with the hope of eventually taking over the practice.

By the late 1940s there was growing concern that newly graduated doctors lacked the necessary experience to begin independent

practice.[11] Following extensive debate, a compulsory 1-year programme of supervised practice in hospital (the pre-registration year)
was introduced in 1953. On graduation, the doctor received provi-
sional registration with the GMC. Full registration, and with it the
right to independent practice, could only take place after successful
completion of pre-registration house jobs.

As medical practice became more complex, postgraduate training
became, from necessity, more structured. Training posts were formally recognised by the NHS and the incumbents received a salary.
Training was experiential, with little formal educational input, and
by the 1960s much of the medical care of patients in hospital was
being delivered by doctors in training. There were inevitable tensions
between the educational needs of the doctors and the pressures of
service delivery.

Major reform of the system was necessary, and in 1993 a review
under the chairmanship of the Chief Medical Officer, Sir Kenneth
Calman, recommended formalisation of specialty training. Medical
specialties and sub-specialties were defined and the relevant training
programmes for each sub-specialty were agreed.[12]

The re-organisation of training at specialty level highlighted the
lack of organisation of training a more junior level – the senior house
officer grade[13] – and led in turn to a restructuring of the whole of
postgraduate training that acknowledged the new challenges presented by the increasing sub-specialisation of medicine. In 2005
the pre-registration house officer grade was replaced by a 2-year
Foundation Programme comprising six 4-month-long attachments
in a variety of specialties.[14] The Foundation Programme introduced
more formal approaches to education and assessment into the
early postgraduate experience. Full registration with the GMC still
takes place after 1 year of postgraduate training, but trainees cannot
progress to the next stage of training until they have completed the
Foundation Programme. There has been discussion about progress
being determined by the attainment of defined competencies rather
than being time based, but so far this has not been implemented
(*see* Chapter 3).

FROM SOLO PRACTITIONER TO TEAM MEMBER

The common assumption in the medical codes appears to be that
the physician will act within a one-to-one relationship with a patient
who has initiated the contact between the two. This reflects the
predominant pattern of medical practice in historical times. While

at some times and in some places physicians may have practised as members of a clearly defined group (for example, as priests in temples to Asclepius or Apollo), more often they were independent practitioners living in the community that they served and delivering medical care when called upon to do so. Even when patients were treated in hospital, they were cared for by their individual doctor (as is still the case in private healthcare systems).

As training became more formalised, trainees were associated with individual doctors, and a group of trainees of differing levels of experience attached to a single consultant were known as a 'firm'. They acted as a team for the delivery of care to that consultant's patients but they were largely independent of external support, except when the patient's illness required referral to another specialty. Other healthcare professions existed, but their roles were well defined and did not overlap with those of the doctor.

The situation is now very different. As specialties have multiplied, multidisciplinary care has become the norm. Patients with breast cancer are no longer treated by a general surgeon who performs an operation and carries out follow-up. Instead, their case will be discussed at a multidisciplinary team meeting and their care will be managed by a specialist breast surgeon, a medical oncologist, and a radiation oncologist, with active advice from a specialist breast radiologist and a specialist breast pathologist. The patient will receive support from a breast care nurse and may have advice from a physiotherapist with a special interest in patients with breast disease. Similar arrangements are in place for a wide range of other conditions.

The multidisciplinary team itself is governed by national guidelines and local protocols. These are developed as a consensus of the views of expert clinicians drawing on the best available evidence from the literature. There is increasing pressure for clinicians to conform to such guidelines. This has the advantage of ensuring consistency in management across all patients with a given condition but it carries the risk that individual patients may receive treatment that is inappropriate to them.

As physicians have narrowed the focus of their individual expertise, other professions have extended their role. Nurse practitioners now undertake a range of tasks that were previously restricted to doctors, including acting as independent practitioners in primary care with rights and competences to make diagnoses and to prescribe a wide range of drugs.[15] Consultant physiotherapists can diagnose musculoskeletal disorders and formulate management plans. Radiographers not only perform radiological investigations but also report the results. This has inevitably raised questions about the precise role of the doctor within the healthcare team.

The GMC in *Tomorrow's Doctors 2009* requires that medical students should, on graduation, be able to 'learn and work effectively in a multidisciplinary team'.[16] More specifically, they should 'demonstrate the ability to . . . undertake various team roles including leadership and the ability to accept leadership from others'.[16] There is no guidance on how the balance between displaying leadership and accepting the leadership of others is to be determined.

Tomorrow's Doctors also suggests that doctors have particular responsibility for 'using their ability to . . . analyse complex and difficult situations'.[16] At first sight this distinguishes the function of the doctor from that of other health professionals, but on reflection it raises questions about who is responsible for identifying a case as 'complex and difficult'. How and at what point would a doctor become involved?

The shape and function of healthcare teams continue to evolve. Education and training for healthcare is rather more slowly adapting to the changes. The regulation, and with it the self-identification of the professions involved, will also have to change.

OTHER MEDICAL ROLES

Although the commonest image of the doctor centres on patient care, other roles are important. In 1846, William Duncan was appointed as Medical Officer for Health in Liverpool, with responsibility for improving public health in the city.[17] Two years later, the importance of public health was recognised in the Public Health Act of 1848.[18] In the same year, John Simon was appointed as Medical Officer for Health in the City of London. By the beginning of the twentieth century every municipal authority in the United Kingdom had a Medical Officer for Health. The early practitioners often held appointments as physicians or surgeons in addition to their duties as public health specialists. John Snow, who is regarded as the father of epidemiology, as a result of his identification of the Broad Street Pump as the source of a cholera epidemic in London in 1854, was a physician at Westminster Hospital and was one of the earliest exponents of anaesthesia with ether and chloroform; he personally administered anaesthesia to Queen Victoria for the birth of two of her children.[19]

As the discipline of public health developed, its practitioners became more specialised and eventually formed the Faculty of Public

Health within the Royal College of Physicians in 1972.[20] Fellowship of the Faculty is open to non-physicians and a substantial proportion of the senior public health workforce is non-medical, once again raising questions about the exact nature of what it means to be a physician.

As health services have become more bureaucratic, the doctor's role in managing the service has changed. The concept of doctors in management roles is not new. Before the inception of the NHS, physician superintendents effectively functioning as chief executive officers led many hospitals. Within current structures it is rare for chief executive officers of healthcare organisations to be physicians, but in UK health organisations one of the executive directors will normally be a physician. The medical director usually continues to work part-time as a clinician and is supported by a number of clinical directors below board level who are responsible for managing the delivery of service within their group of disciplines. The growing complexity of these roles has led to an increasing number of doctors choosing to study for qualifications in management including Master of Business Administration degrees (*see* Chapter 5).

All doctors have a professional duty to be involved in educating and training the next generation (*see* Chapter 11). However, over the past 25 years the role of medical educator has become more clearly delineated. Like medical managers, most educators continue to practise clinically but they have developed special expertise in the science and technology of education. They have their own professional organisations and specialist training, including master's degrees and doctorates in education, and are responsible for the design and management of training programmes at all levels, from undergraduate to continuing professional development. However, the delivery of the majority of training is still dependent on ordinary practising clinicians.

CONCLUSION

The medical profession is in a state of flux. Traditional roles are changing and new roles are emerging. The current generation of practitioners, in whatever role they occupy, still self-identify as physicians and trace their lineage back through a gallery of notable predecessors to Hippocrates and beyond. The nature of future roles and self-identity of the profession and how it will interact with other health professionals is still unclear. We live in interesting times.

REFERENCES

1. Tate. Sir Luke Fildes, *The Doctor*, exhibited 1891. Available at: www.tate.org. uk/art/artworks/fildes-the-doctor-n01522 (accessed 13 June 2012).
2. Cross M. Show us the data: why clinical outcomes matter. *BMJ.* 2012; 344: e66.
3. Turner J, Kelly B. Emotional dimensions of chronic disease. *West J Med.* 2000; 172(2): 124–8.
4. *Medical Generalism: why expertise in whole person medicine matters.* Royal College of General Practitioners: London; 2012.
5. Perper JA, Cina SJ. Perfect intentions, imperfect people. In: Perper JA, Cina SJ. *When Doctors Kill: who, why and how.* New York, NY: Springer Science & Business Media; 2010. pp. 9–14.
6. 'Emeritus'. *A Letter on Medical Registration and the Condition of the Medical Corporations.* London: Jackson; 1852.
7. Medical Act 1858. Available at: www.legislation.gov.uk/ukpga/Vict/21-22/90/ enacted (accessed 27 July 2012).
8. Smith J. *Fifth Report – Safeguarding Patients: lessons from the past proposals for the future.* 2004. Command Paper Cm 6394. Available at: www.shipman-inquiry. org.uk/fifthreport.asp (accessed 27 July 2012).
9. General Medical Council. *Information for Licensed Doctors.* Available at: www. gmc-uk.org/doctors/revalidation/12382.asp (accessed 13 January 2013).
10. Flexner A. *Medical Education in the United States and Canada: a report to the Carnegie Foundation for the Advancement of Teaching* reproduced in bulletin of the World Health Organization. 2002; 80(7): 594–602.
11. The training of doctors: report by the Goodenough Committee [editorial]. *Br Med J.* 1944; 22(4359): 121–3.
12. Department of Health. *Hospital Doctors: training for the future. The report of the working group on specialist medical training.* London: HMSO; 1993.
13. Dillner L. Senior house officers: the lost tribes. *BMJ.* 1993; 307(6918): 1549–51.
14. UK Foundation Programme Office. *The Foundation Programme Reference Guide 2012.* Cardiff: UK Foundation Programme Office; 2012.
15. www.nursepractitioner.org.uk
16. General Medical Council. *Tomorrow's Doctors 2009.* London: GMC; 2009.
17. Halliday S. Duncan of Liverpool: Britain's first medical officer. *J Med Biogr.* 2003; 11(3): 142–9.
18. Calman K. The 1848 Public Health Act and its relevance to improving public health in England today. *BMJ.* 1998; 317(7158): 596–8.
19. Frerichs R. *John Snow.* Los Angeles: Department of Epidemiology, University of California, Los Angeles; 2009. Available at: www.ph.ucla.edu/epi/snow/ encyclopediasummaryfrerichs.html (accessed 25 July 2012).
20. www.fph.org.uk

CHAPTER 2

The changing working environment: work patterns

Bernard Brett and Susan Miles

INTRODUCTION

The environment in which doctors work is constantly changing, and the rate of change is increasing. Over recent years the environmental changes that have impacted on medical practice include many aspects, such as those of a technological, organisational, managerial and educational nature, and also include reductions in hours worked and alterations in patterns of work. In this chapter we will discuss key changes to working patterns in both secondary and primary care.

SECONDARY CARE

Both the New Deal for Junior Doctors 1991, a package of measures designed to improve the working conditions of junior doctors including limiting working hours, and the European Working Time Directive (enacted into UK law as the Working Time Regulations) have had a profound effect on the working patterns of doctors. This has led to changes in the total number of hours worked on average, the duration of any single shift worked by each junior doctor and the minimum breaks between and during shifts. The resulting alterations made to rotas have in turn affected the structure and function of medical teams and how care is delivered by them to patients.

Historically, for hospital doctors the core working unit was a team of doctors, often called a 'firm', led by a consultant. This team tended to share the same working pattern, with all members sharing on-call days and being responsible for the same group of inpatients and outpatients. All members of the team would be resident (i.e. on site) during on-call periods, with the exception of the consultant and sometimes, when the firm included one, the senior registrar. Depending upon the precise make-up of the team, the registrar or senior registrar would provide much of the day-to-day leadership, support and training and especially out of hours. Each doctor would look for direct support from the member of the team directly above them, as well as peer support from colleagues at the same level in other firms, and in turn support the member/s of the team directly below them.

This firm structure, with the associated working pattern, meant there was a high level of understanding of one another's strengths, weaknesses, training needs and personality. When this medical team was working at its best, all members of staff felt supported and there was a genuine sense of camaraderie and team spirit. Training was facilitated as a result of this high level of understanding, and also because the more senior doctor would gain a genuine benefit from enhancing the skills and knowledge of more junior colleagues, as this would mean they could competently deal with ever more complex cases. Sickness levels tended to be very low, probably at least in part as a result of a sense of loyalty to the team, with team members not wanting to make things difficult for their colleagues.

Continuity of patient care was of a very high level. Most patients were clerked in by a member of a firm (usually the most junior doctor) and then remained under the same team of doctors for the duration of the stay, regardless of where the available beds were.

However, there were also significant disadvantages to such patterns of work. The average number of hours worked was usually over 70 hours per week, and doctors were often on-call for continuous periods of 48, 72 or even 80 hours or more at a time (weekends on-call for many doctors started on a Friday morning and finished on a Monday, early evening). The intensity of work was variable; for some teams it would be the usual expectation that most or all members of the team would manage to get at least 6–8 hours' sleep, with either no or very few interruptions on most nights. However, other teams did suffer from high workloads overnight. On-call rotas of 1 in 3 or 1 in 4 (meaning that the team would be on-call, providing emergency cover, including out-of-hours (OOH) cover, for a 24-hour period every 3 or 4 days while working normal working days (e.g. 8 a.m.–5.30/6 p.m.) on the intervening days), with prospective cover for leave (for periods of planned leave, the doctor would be responsible for swapping his or her on-call), were relatively common. On-call rotas in some specialist fields were particularly onerous, with a frequency of 1 in 2.

Clearly, these patterns of work, especially for those specialties with a greater intensity of work, which often lasted for the first 10 years or more of a doctor's career did cause personal stress and affected family life in the case of some doctors. Junior doctors did, however, gain valuable experience, having been directly involved in the care of a very large number of patients, with a high level of continuity of care and having to take on considerable responsibility early in their career.

The recent changes in working hours described here have led to many hospital specialties moving to a shift pattern of working. In addition, many have moved to a ward-based model of care. In full-shift rotas each doctor will usually work a maximum of 12½ hours and usually a minimum of 8 hours per shift. In addition, rotas include a series of nightshifts for 2–7 continuous nights. Nightshifts are often incorporated into a system of working called Hospital at Night (discussed in more detail shortly). In ward-based care models, the junior doctor and consultant who first admit a patient will usually pass over the responsibility of care for the patient to another team as soon as the patient moves to an inpatient ward. Each consultant team will then be responsible for all the patients on a particular ward or on certain bays in a particular ward. Where possible, the patient is preferentially moved to a ward covered by a team of doctors and nurses with the specialty interest most appropriate to that patient's needs.

In most hospitals, for most specialties the rotas for junior doctors are not completely aligned to those for other members of the team, or, indeed, to the consultant of that team; often there is no alignment and they only work together while on-call occasionally by chance. This means that when on-call, each junior doctor will usually work with a different group of doctors depending upon their pattern of work for a particular week. The consequences of these changes are that there is a significantly greater need for high-quality written and verbal communication to ensure optimal patient care; in the old model the continuity of care provided by all members of the team meant that there was far less need for handovers. In addition, high-quality communication is also important to ensure the training needs for junior doctors are met (*see* Chapter 3).

Research following the introduction of rota-based shift working and consequent reorganisation of working teams indicated doctor-held concerns regarding less continuity of patient care. Doctors were concerned about 'shift mentality', where doctors just leave at the end of their shift, and some doctors actively worked harder to avoid handing over tasks to the next shift. It also illustrated the importance of good-quality handovers, to prevent patient care becoming even more disjointed. It found improved specialist registrar-led care for patients at nights and weekends, but it also found a lack of ownership of clinical problems by junior doctors, and continuity of patient care at post-take ward rounds had devolved to consultants.[1,2]

Research evidence suggests that patient care (as assessed by measures such as length of stay, number and episodes of readmissions, death during admission) has not been affected by changes to working patterns as a result of compliance to the European Working Time Directive.[3,4] Quality of care was generally regarded as having improved as a result of doctors now being more alert.[1] Some doctors felt that their enjoyment of the job had dropped since changing to shift working and that their quality of life outside of work had reduced, as it was harder to sort family life and they only went home to sleep.[1] Research has also found evidence of more sick leave among junior doctors, which was attributed to a loss of group cohesiveness.[3]

Hospital at Night

In the traditional National Health Service (NHS) model, on-call specialist teams generally covered patient care at night. There would be a variable number of specialty teams, depending upon the size of the hospital and the number of secondary and tertiary services the hospital provided. These teams tended to work in relative isolation. General practitioners (GPs) and the accident and emergency department would refer potential admissions to the team they felt would be most appropriate. The team would then accept, reject, or accept and then refer on each patient. Once admitted to an inpatient area, the team who had admitted the patient usually covered the patient until discharge.

Hospital at Night (H@N) describes an approach to providing night cover in hospitals using multidisciplinary teams with the ability to call in specialist expertise if required. H@N was introduced to reduce reliance on junior doctors for providing night cover while improving doctors' quality of working life and patient care.[5] These teams vary from hospital to hospital, but they usually have one or more individuals who coordinate all staff covering the night. A system of bleep filtering is commonly used, where the coordinator will bleep the most appropriate member of the team as needed, rather than doctors being bleeped constantly by different people. Most members of the H@N team work in a more generic way: junior doctors might, for example, be tasked to cover the inpatient areas, and they would assist with the clinical management of any patient regardless of the specialty responsible for managing the patient's care during the day. This could mean that a medical junior doctor might be the first doctor to see a patient under the orthopaedic surgeons who had developed an acute problem overnight. H@N teams usually include one or more nurses. H@N nurses have been trained to undertake some of the tasks that doctors would have traditionally undertaken. These tasks include procedures such as taking blood or blood cultures, the insertion of intravenous cannulas, performing electrocardiograms and inserting urinary catheters. They would also often be trained to undertake some degree of clinical assessment, management and limited prescribing. Each H@N team is made up of members of staff who do not usually work together regularly during the day and who may have limited knowledge – at least at the start of a new rota cycle – of one another's strengths and weaknesses.

There has been little research on the impact of H@N on patient safety and staff satisfaction since the largely positive evaluation of the pilot projects.[5] There is evidence that the introduction of H@N has led to more frequent patient review by senior staff and has reduced adverse patient outcomes.[6] Junior doctors report beneficial exposure to acute clinical problems at night,[2] and research indicates that there are suitable opportunities to achieve Foundation training competencies while working on the H@N team.[7] However, while some members of the H@N team appreciate the opportunity to experience a variety of specialties while covering other areas, other members are dissatisfied with the loss of time in their own specialty.[1,2]

H@N has helped to deliver safe care while enabling the reduction of hours of work for junior doctors. This system of work is more efficient and has many advantages but it has also created challenges. Healthcare organisations need to ensure that measures are put in place to provide appropriate training for team members and to refine these systems to the benefit of patients and staff, including doctors.

PRIMARY CARE

Traditionally GPs were self-employed contractors who were, individually, responsible for the care of their patients 24 hours a day. However, the working patterns of GPs have undergone considerable change in recent years; perhaps most notably with regard to OOH working (i.e. weekends; public and bank holidays; 6.30 p.m.–8.00 a.m., weekdays). The National Health Service (Primary Care) Act 1997 and the nationally agreed 2004 General Medical Services (GMS) contract recognised the need for more balance between work and home for GPs and, as such, provided increased opportunity for practices to control their workload and to have greater working flexibility in a number of areas. Such changes have led to a greater role for practice nurses and practice managers, and to the increasing need for GPs to work collaboratively with other doctors and a variety of other professions.

The 1997 Act led to a growing number of GPs being employed on salaried contracts. These contracts gave GPs more ability to choose when and where to work, as they were not financially tied into a practice partnership, and they offered freedom from administrative, financial and other managerial responsibilities. Early research indicated that salaried doctors were more satisfied with their hours of work and were less stressed regarding administrative and managerial responsibilities – including worrying about paperwork, finances, patient complaints or litigation, and finding locums to cover absences – than non-salaried GPs.[8] They were also less stressed about activities associated with OOH service provision. However, they were more stressed about professional isolation. There was no difference in overall job satisfaction.[8] It has been argued that the introduction of salaried posts has appealed to a subset of GPs who did not fit well into the traditional model of self-employed partners in a practice, which may increase job satisfaction and workforce participation among these GPs.[9]

The new GMS contract afforded GPs more choice in deciding the range of services they would provide. While all practices are required to provide 'essential' services for their patients, they have the option to provide 'additional' services (e.g. cervical screening, vaccinations and immunisations, maternity medical services). This enabled GPs to develop specialties in particular areas, gain extra income by providing these services, or to temporarily or permanently opt out of providing these services.

The nature of the contract was changed, such that the GMS contract was now between the primary care organisation (PCO) (e.g. primary care trusts) and the practice, rather than with individual GPs (the contract for GP practices will be between the National Care Board and GPs). This, in combination with a change to the payment structure, allowed practices to invest in infrastructure including premises, information technology and the ability to employ the staff they require to meet local needs. It also allowed for further flexibility in the individual's working patterns.

The new GMS contract also introduced a quality and outcomes framework (QuOF) based on research evidence, whereby practices achieve points for the quality of their care in various domains and these points translate into financial reward. In this way, practices are directly rewarded for providing high-quality care to patients (*see* Chapter 6). Those practices working under a personal medical services (PMS) contract (where services are locally agreed with the PCO) are also able to participate in the national QuOF scheme.

The new GMS contract transferred responsibility for arranging 24-hour cover to PCOs, allowing GPs to opt out of providing, and the responsibility for arranging, OOH care if they so wished. PMS contract practices can also transfer responsibility for OOH. Increasing demand for 24-hour care by patients and desire among GPs for a better work-home balance had already led to a variety of models of OOH service provision before the new GMS contract, including the following: GPs providing OOH care themselves, joining a practice rota (where GPs at the same practice take it in turns to provide care for patients registered at the practice), joining a GP cooperative (where a group of practices worked together to provide cover for all their patients) and utilising a commercial deputising service. Further developments in this area led to the formation of primary care centres where the patients would come to the doctor (as opposed to home visits to the patient), NHS walk-in centres, and partnerships between local NHS Direct 24-hour telephone sites and GP cooperatives to provide triage and subsequent telephone or face-to-face consultations.[10] The implications of OOH service provision on GP training and patient and GP satisfaction are wide-ranging and will be discussed further.

With GP trainers opting out of OOH service provision, there was some concern that GPs in training (GP registrars) would have limited opportunities to develop essential skills in clinical decision-making in complex settings where the patient is unfamiliar, previous notes are unavailable and the physical situation may be inadequate.[11] Research investigating the experiences of GP registrars with their OOH training indicated that they were positive about their induction, their educational experiences, their supervision, and organising their training; however, they were less positive about the record sheets and workbooks they had to complete during training.[12] Further research is needed to ascertain the long-term effect of this change in training for GP registrars.

Patient experiences with OOH service provision have been mixed but chiefly positive. The most recent GP Patient Survey (2011–12) indicated that only 58% of patients knew how to contact an OOH GP service if needed.[13] However, generally those who had contacted the service in the past 6 months found it easy to contact, most felt it took the right amount of time to receive care, the majority had trust and confidence in the OOH clinician and most thought their experience was good. Despite this, there was a significant minority who had not had a satisfactory experience, suggesting that more work is needed to improve the quality of OOH care.

Satisfaction is strongly influenced by waiting times in the following areas: time for the call to be answered, to receive a call back, for the home visit or appointment at the centre. Aspects of the consultation also influence satisfaction, including the length of consultation time, quality of communication with the OOH doctor (including listening to the patient, explaining clearly, not talking down to the patient), and whether appropriate advice and medication are given. Other issues that can affect satisfaction include whether prescribed medication can be accessed out of hours; provision of information about after-care, including under what circumstances to contact the GP for follow-up; the manner of the gatekeeper; and efficiency of triage (e.g. having to answer the same questions for the telephone operator, nurse and doctor; struggling to get past the gatekeeper to the doctor). Getting to the centre for an appointment was affected by factors such as the large area covered by the OOH service provider (meaning that the distance to travel is long), availability of own transport, appropriate signposting at the centre, feeling too ill to travel, and safety concerns about taking a young child out at night alone. Some patients also had concerns about continuity of care, because of the OOH service provider not knowing their medical history and ongoing investigations.[14–16]

Regarding the experiences of GPs themselves with the new GMS contract generally, and changes to OOH provisions specifically, a postal survey of GPs conducted immediately prior to and 18 months after the 2004 GMS contract was introduced found that job satisfaction had increased in a number of areas (including remuneration and hours of work) and job pressure (particularly related to night visits and 24-hour responsibility for patients) had decreased. Furthermore, while GPs felt that their professional autonomy had decreased and their clinical and administrative workloads had increased, they also felt that overall quality of care and quality of preventive care and care of chronic diseases had increased since the introduction of the new contract.[17] More recently, interviews indicated that while salaried GPs had some concerns about less continuity of care for patients because of opting out of OOH and nurses doing day-to-day QuOF work, they did feel that the QuOF had led to improved and standardised clinical care across the profession, and they felt that they had more flexibility regarding their work-life balance. While noting a difference in pay with their employing GPs, the salaried GPs did feel that this fairly reflected differences in responsibility.[18]

Even before GPs were able to opt out of OOH service provision, there was some concern that the introduction of GP cooperatives might put additional pressure on accident and emergency departments, but research conducted has not borne this out.[19,20] However, there has been little research in this area following the 2004 GMS contract, and what research there is indicates that the impact of changes to provision of primary care OOH services on secondary care is difficult to measure.[21] The biggest pressure facing secondary and tertiary care is the rising number of admissions of elderly patients with complex medical problems (usually multiple long-term conditions) often exacerbated by social factors. The experiences of secondary care are that many patients end up being sent to hospital by the OOH services when their own GP would probably have managed them in the community.

Safety is another factor to consider. Negative patient outcomes have resulted from OOH providers failing to assess the competence of clinical staff, including the language skills of overseas doctors. Following the death of a gentleman because of an overdose of opiates administered by a locum doctor who normally practised in Germany, a review of the local commissioning and provision of out-of-hours services made a number of recommendations to make OOH service more effective and safe.[22]

RECOMMENDATIONS

The change in working patterns brought about by the reduced working hours and rota-based shift working discussed here means that doctors require additional skills to operate efficiently in their current working environment. Consequently, the following recommendations are made to optimise safe practice and quality of working life.

➤ Doctors need to be trained in and to pay attention to their communication skills, both with patients and with other healthcare professionals. High-quality oral and written handover is essential to maintain patient care with changing shifts and medical responsibility for each patient.

➤ Doctors must increasingly focus on communicating their competencies and training needs and understanding those of others, particularly in H@N teams, to ensure high-quality care delivery and training.

➤ Junior doctors need to take ownership of their learning and to make good use of private study time, timetabled teaching sessions (even possibly when they are not on shift) and clinical experiences both within and beyond their specialty when working H@N.

➤ Junior doctors need to ensure that regular meetings with their supervisors occur, even if they are not frequently working on the same shifts.

➤ Doctors need to be well organised, they need to prioritise tasks and they need to manage their workload to ensure that they are working productively and are not placing an inappropriate burden of work on their colleagues when they go off shift.

➤ Senior doctors need to encourage team building to support a professional commitment to colleagues and patients.

➤ Leadership skills need to become part of medical school training in order to ensure that doctors are prepared to lead the diverse teams they will be responsible for during their careers. Management skills are also increasingly important (*see* Chapter 5).

➤ Each doctor in training needs to seek and be given high-quality career advice to enable them to make the best choices in this changing healthcare environment.

REFERENCES

1. Bamford N, Bamford D. The effect of a full shift system on doctors. *J Health Organ Manag.* 2008; **22**(3): 223–37.
2. Jones GJ, Vanderpump MP, Easton M, *et al.* Achieving compliance with the European Working Time Directive in a large teaching hospital: a strategic approach. *Clin Med.* 2004; **4**(5): 427–30.
3. McIntyre HF, Winfield S, Te HS, *et al.* Implementation of the European Working Time Directive in an NHS trust: impact on patient care and junior doctor welfare. *Clin Med.* 2010; **10**(2): 134–7.
4. Collum J, Harrop J, Stokes M, *et al.* Patient safety and quality of care continue to improve in NHS North West following early implementation of the European Working Time Directive. *QJM.* 2010; **103**(12): 929–40.

5. Department of Health. *The Implementation and Impact of Hospital at Night Pilot Projects: an evaluation report.* London: Department of Health; 2005.

6. Beckett DJ, Gordon CF, Paterson R, *et al.* Improvement in out-of-hours outcomes following the implementation of Hospital at Night. *QJM.* 2009; **102**(8): 539–46.

7. Gallagher P, McLean P, Campbell R, *et al.* Medical training and the hospital at night: an oxymoron? *Med Educ.* 2009; **43**(11): 1056–61.

8. Gosden T, Williams J, Petchey R, *et al.* Salaried contracts in UK general practice: a study of job satisfaction and stress. *J Health Serv Res Policy.* 2002; **7**(1): 26–33.

9. Ding A, Hann M, Sibbald B. Profile of English salaried GPs: labour mobility and practice performance. *Br J Gen Pract.* 2008; **58**(546): 20–5.

10. Department of Health. *Raising Standards for Patients: new partnerships in out-of-hours care.* London: HMSO; 2000.

11. Campbell JL, Clay JH. Out-of-hours care: do we? *Br J Gen Pract.* 2010; **60**(572): 155–7.

12. Lewis GH, Sullivan MJ, Tanner R, *et al.* Exploring the perceptions of out-of-hours training for GP registrars in Wales. *Educ Prim Care.* 2009; **20**(3): 152–8.

13. www.gp-patient.co.uk

14. Poole R, Gamper A, Porter A, *et al.* Exploring patients' self-reported experiences of out-of-hours primary care and their suggestions for improvement: a qualitative study. *Fam Pract.* 2011; **28**(2): 210–19.

15. Kinnersley P, Egbunike JN, Kelly M, *et al.* The need to improve the interface between in-hours and out-of-hours GP care, and between out-of-hours care and self-care. *Fam Pract.* 2010; **27**(6): 664–72.

16. Egbunike JN, Shaw C, Porter A, *et al.* Streamline triage and manage user expectations: lessons from a qualitative study of GP out-of-hours services. *Br J Gen Pract.* 2010; **60**(572): e83–97.

17. Whalley D, Gravelle H, Sibbald B. Effect of the new contract on GPs' working lives and perceptions of quality of care: a longitudinal survey. *Br J Gen Pract.* 2008; **58**(546): 8–14.

18. Cheraghi-Sohi S, McDonald R, Harrison S, *et al.* Experience of contractual change in UK general practice: a qualitative study of salaried GPs. *Br J Gen Pract.* 2012; **62**(597): e282–7.

19. Pickin DM, O'Cathain A, Fall M, *et al.* The impact of a general practice co-operative on accident and emergency services, patient satisfaction and GP satisfaction. *Fam Pract.* 2004; **21**(2): 180–2.

20. O'Keeffe N. The effect of a new general practice out-of-hours co-operative on a county hospital accident and emergency department. *Ir J Med Sci.* 2008; **177**(4): 367–70.

21. Thompson C, Hayhurst C, Boyle A. How have changes to out-of-hours primary care services since 2004 affected emergency department attendances at a UK District General Hospital? A longitudinal study. *Emerg Med J.* 2010; **27**(1): 22–5.

22. Colin-Fromé D, Field S. *General Practice Out-of-Hours Services: project to consider and assess current arrangements.* London: Department of Health; 2010.

CHAPTER 3

Changes in postgraduate medical education and training

Joanne Kellett and Veena Rodrigues

INTRODUCTION

Postgraduate medical education and training in the United Kingdom is being delivered in a constantly changing environment. The key drivers for change include changing social demographics, evolving trainee needs and expectations, and political and health service developments.[1,2]

The NHS Plan of 2000 included the commitment to increase the number of consultants and general practitioners (GPs) in order to better respond to rising patient demands.[3] There was also a call to modernise the senior house officer (SHO) grade in response to the view that there were several problems with the training, as doctors had few defined educational goals with a lack of curriculum and assessments, no clear educational or career pathways, no limit to time spent in the grade and a lack of distinction between service and training.[4]

One of the most significant developments in education and training was the launch of Modernising Medical Careers (MMC) in 2003, which was introduced by the government as a means of increasing the quality of care for patients through a new structure of postgraduate medical education and training.[5] MMC was introduced to provide a transparent career path for doctors while also improving quality of patient care. Trainees would be assured of a high quality of training, improved formal supervision and continuous development of acquired competencies. A higher proportion of patient care would be delivered by a skilled workforce with less reliance for service delivery on those still in training.

This chapter will focus on changes made in recent years to post-graduate education and training. It will explore how doctors progress in their training following medical school and it will highlight how curricula, supervision and assessments have changed and the impact that these changes have had on the profession.

CHANGES IN TRAINING PATHWAYS

It was intended that locally delivered training should meet national standards set by the Postgraduate and Medical Education and Training Board, through better structured and managed programmes using competency-based curricula. This resulted in a change to the structure of medical training: in 2005 the new Foundation Programme, a 2-year programme (F1 and F2) of supervised training, replaced the old system of pre-registration house officer and SHO. Foundation doctors who have successfully completed F1 training are eligible to apply to the General Medical Council (GMC) for full registration to practise in the United Kingdom. Following completion of Foundation training, junior doctors move on to competitive entry into limited numbers of specialist and general practice 'run-through training' programmes (3–7 years) or into fixed-term specialist training.

Generic standards for specialty training, including general practice, are currently prescribed nationally by the GMC, following its merger with the Postgraduate and Medical Education and Training Board in 2010.[6] Delivery of training is quality assured against these standards by the GMC. It is expected that this single regulatory responsibility from undergraduate medical education through post-graduate training to clinical practice until retirement will result in consistent expectations and standards. Further changes are expected as part of the UK government's health reforms, with the functions of postgraduate deaneries taken over by local provider skills networks (local education and training boards) constituted by National Health Service (NHS) healthcare providers when strategic health authorities are abolished in 2013.[7]

THE FOUNDATION PROGRAMME

Following undergraduate medical training, graduates progress on to the 2-year structured Foundation Programme. It is designed to give trainees a range of general experience to enable them to take on supervised responsibility for patient care, before choosing an area of medicine in which to specialise. The purpose of the first year is to strengthen and consolidate the knowledge, skills and competence acquired during undergraduate training in order to be fully registered as a medical practitioner with the GMC.[8] The second year focuses on learning to care for the acutely ill patient and the development of generic professional skills such as team working, time management and communication skills.[9] Unlike the old system, F1 trainees move straight on to the second year without having to apply for posts.

Foundation training, implemented by postgraduate deaneries through 25 UK Foundation schools, follows a national curriculum (revised in 2012) and ensures that trainees have opportunities for exposure to a range of specialties through six 4-month placements over the 2-year programme, using workplace-based assessments and feedback to inform professional development.[10] Across the United Kingdom in 2010–11, the top three specialties experienced by F1 doctors were general surgery (83.4%), general (internal) medicine (64.4%) and geriatric medicine (23.7%). The top three specialties experienced by F2 doctors were general practice (42.0%), emergency medicine (41.0%) and general (internal) medicine (20.4%).[11] In August 2011, 97.5% of F1 doctors and 96.4% of F2 doctors successfully completed their respective Foundation years. Where the career destination was known, 71% of F2 doctors were appointed to specialty training in the United Kingdom.

SPECIALTY TRAINING

Over the past 2 decades, there have been several changes to postgraduate medical education designed to strengthen and improve the quality of higher specialist training in the United Kingdom. Following publication of the report of the working group on specialist medical training in 1993, a new specialist registrar training programme was developed and rolled out to all specialties by March 1997.[12,13] Since August 2007 the specialty registrar replaces the specialist registrar and GP registrar. During the F2 year, trainees are required to choose a specialty that they will focus on during the next stage of postgraduate training. There are two types of programmes, depending on the specialty: (1) 'run-through' training (3–7 years), where progression between levels is automatic as long as competency requirements are met, and (2) 'uncoupled' training programmes including 2 or 3 years of core specialty training followed by open competition for higher specialty training posts. In 2010 the three specialties that had the most trainees were anaesthetics, paediatrics, and obstetrics and gynaecology.[14]

RECRUITMENT PROCESS

Recruitment to the Foundation Programme follows a national recruitment process, with applications for final-year medical students in the United Kingdom made through completion of an online application form. Application forms are scored by Foundation schools, and applicants are allocated to schools and programmes based on rankings of their scores and preferences.[9]

Applications to enter specialist training programmes are coordinated nationally, either by a lead deanery or by one of the Royal Colleges on behalf of all the English deaneries. Applications follow an online process, with a single application form per specialty specifying preferred deaneries for training.[15] Currently applicants receive offers directly from each deanery. However, from 2013 onwards, all first offers will be coordinated electronically using the UK Offers System, which has been used successfully in Scotland for coordinating offers for the past few years. This will enable applicants to accept, reject or hold first offers until all offers have been issued.

Eligibility criteria and nationally agreed person specifications for individual specialties are also made available online for each specialty, along with competition ratios to inform potential applicants of the demand for each specialty by deanery.[16] Application forms are scored by recruitment offices against person specifications, and top-scoring applicants are invited to assessments (such as numeric and verbal reasoning and situational judgement tests) and/or interviews; the structure and content of these might differ across deaneries and specialties. Posts or appointments to training programmes are offered to the highest-ranked individuals according to their stated preferences.

TRAINING CONTENT, DELIVERY AND ASSESSMENT

Current postgraduate training is designed to build on undergraduate medical education, through application of knowledge and skills gained in the workplace setting with increasing degrees of responsibility, and under the supervision of experienced doctors. Where previously the curricula focused primarily on teaching medical techniques and procedures, the new curricula cover a wider range of skills and competencies such as communication skills, team working, multiprofessional practice, leadership, time management, partnership with patients, quality and safety improvements and the use of evidence and data.[10,14]

Standards for training prescribed by the GMC apply to Foundation training and all specialties including general practice, and the delivery of training by postgraduate deaneries is quality assured against these standards.[6] Training is expected to occur under supervision proportionate to the level of competence of the trainee in the interests of patient safety, and preparing doctors for independent practice and lifelong learning. Training programmes are expected to deliver and assess the requirements of the approved curriculum.

Trainees are expected to acquire knowledge, skills and experience through an appropriate workload, effective supervision and feedback, appropriate learning opportunities and personal support. This is facilitated through regular meetings to discuss progress and achievement of learning needs with designated educational supervisors. Assessment of clinical performance through workplace-based assessments (WBAs) also enables evaluation of performance in context and permits assessors to provide constructive feedback to enhance clinical performance where necessary.

WBAs used currently in Foundation and specialist training include direct observation of clinical activities through direct observation of procedural skills (DOPs) and the Mini-Clinical Evaluation Exercise (mini-CEX); discussion of clinical cases through case-based discussion (CBD); a form of multisource feedback such as a peer assessment tool (mini-PAT) or team assessment of behaviour (TAB); and, more recently, a new WBA (developing the clinical teacher) to assess teaching and presentation skills of Foundation doctors.[17]

Assessment from a range of sources is used to certify achievement of competence at the end of the second year of Foundation training. These include direct observation of the doctor's performance, feedback from colleagues, discussions with the doctor, and the doctor's portfolio of evidence.[9]

For specialist trainees, annual reviews of competence and progression are conducted by training programmes and focus on assessment of a portfolio submitted by trainees to evidence achievements against relevant learning outcomes. This enables a panel of assessors to make decisions on trainee progression through training, which includes the identification of trainees in need of additional support at an early stage, as well as a recommendation for the Certificate of Completion of Training for trainees who have successfully completed all training requirements. The Certificate of Completion of Training enables trainees to apply to the GMC for entry to the Specialist or GP Register.[18]

IMPACT OF CHANGES ON TRAINING

A number of key reports have highlighted the need for further improvement to the process of postgraduate education reform.[19-21] An independent review of MMC in 2008 found the experiences of trainees to be variable, with 69% of doctors surveyed reporting that F2 was not an improvement on the SHO post that it had replaced, and two-thirds reporting they felt that Foundation training had not had a positive effect on clinical service delivery.[19] Concerns were also raised about the integration of the F1 year with the final undergraduate year, the validity and robustness of the competency assessments, the length and relevance of F2 placements, and the premature choice of specialty halfway through the F2 year, with fewer than a third of trainees knowing which specialty they wished to pursue at the end of the F1 year. The review found that the policy objective of postgraduate medical training was unclear, with no consensus on the educational principles guiding the training or the role of doctors, and a lack of cohesion in the training structure.

A recent evaluation of the Foundation Programme highlighted several strengths such as the educational infrastructure, national curriculum, regular assessment and feedback, but also some concerns such as the selection process, length of the programme and rotations, lack of flexibility in the programme, tensions between demands of clinical service and requirements for learning and gaps in the curriculum, with insufficient emphasis on the total patient and on long-term conditions.[21] Specific recommendations made to address concerns identified have been addressed in the 2012 revision of the curriculum, which has an added resource section providing external links to relevant material to support the curriculum, including the e-Learning for Healthcare resource developed by the Foundation Programme Office in partnership with the Academy of Medical Royal Colleges.[10] The e-Learning for Healthcare e-learning modules are interactive, map directly to the Foundation curriculum and are designed to enhance existing teaching within Foundation schools.[22]

National trainee surveys in 2010 and 2011 found levels of satisfaction with training improving by year.[23,24] The latest GMC trainee survey of 46 668 doctors found satisfaction with training high (with GP trainees most satisfied and surgical trainees least satisfied), but there were some areas for concern.[24] Medical graduates needed to be better prepared for some aspects of the job when they entered Foundation training; 61% of trainees said they did feel adequately prepared for their first F1 post, compared with 58% in 2010. This finding mirrors other research studies that have reported that improvements are required in preparing graduates for clinical practice, especially around prescribing and practical skills.[21,25-27] Other issues raised included Foundation trainees reporting doing routine work of no educational value and feeling pressured to cope with problems beyond their clinical competence.[24] One study that examined perceptions of Foundation trainees, consultants and senior nurses about the introduction of the Foundation Programme found a mixed response.[28] Certain specialties were seen as offering insufficiently generic experience and consultants were concerned that rotations were too short. Trainees were not able to see cases through because of frequently moving around, and continuity of care was perceived to be provided by nurses and consultants rather than Foundation doctors. The study also found that levels of responsibility varied widely between posts and specialties and, as a result, some F2s reported frustration that they were not given enough responsibility for this stage of their training.

A further concern highlighted among trainees and trainers related to supervision; assessments within the Foundation Programme have placed a new requirement on supervisors and trainers. There were varied experiences reported by trainees regarding supervisory experience in terms of access and lack of regular planned contact. The 2011 trainee survey reported that more feedback was required from senior colleagues and supervisors, as over a quarter of Foundation and specialty trainees said that they never or rarely received informal feedback from a senior clinician, supervisor or senior colleague.[24] Many felt a lack of training, support and supervision, and Foundation trainees raised concerns about the value of electronic portfolio requirements, with only a third reporting that the learning portfolio helped them with their learning needs. A GMC survey of 15 062 trainers also reported concerns about the assessments of trainees, with evidence that WBAs were widely perceived by trainers and trainees to be a 'tick-box exercise' that could mask performance problems.[29] Consultants reported that the service demands made of trainees often meant that they missed out on learning opportunities, and the majority of trainers felt that trainees were less confident and less able to work independently than when they themselves were trained. Similarly, an evaluation of the Foundation Programme found that the assessment of Foundation doctors was considered to be excessive, onerous and not valued.[21] Variation was also reported in the supervision of trainees, the quality of education and learning and the lack of pastoral care. Concerns about inconsistencies in training delivered to postgraduate medical supervisors across Royal Colleges and deaneries, has led to the development of a framework for professional development of postgraduate medical supervisors of doctors in training by the Academy of Medical Educators.[30] The GMC has recently consulted on, and is expected to publish new arrangements for, the recognition and approval of trainers in late 2012 in order to develop a systematic approach to high-quality training similar to that used in general practice.[31]

EUROPEAN WORKING TIME DIRECTIVE

To meet the aim of building greater capacity within the health service, MMC sought to reduce the time that junior doctors spent in their postgraduate training, by focusing on a more focused and structured training programme. In addition, the European Working Time Directive (EWTD) introduced a 48-hour week for junior doctors from August 2009 into UK law. While some evidence from other countries has suggested that restricting working hours to less than 80 a week has had no adverse effects on patient safety and postgraduate training,[32] concerns have remained in the United Kingdom around the impact of the EWTD on the education and training of postgraduate doctors.[14,19,20,28]

There is some evidence that restricted working hours has led to fewer fatigue-related errors and multidisciplinary teams are now often providing services previously provided by trainee doctors, such as phlebotomy, cannulation and basic administrative duties, allowing more time for valuable training activity.[32] However, a review of the impact of the EWTD on the quality of training found increased tensions between service delivery and protected time for education and training. In particular, the main impact has been felt in specialties with high emergency or out-of-hours workloads, where medical trainees were often required to provide patient care when there were gaps in rotas.[20] In a 2011 survey more than 20% of trainees stated that they were not having their training requirements met within the 48-hour week and more than half of Foundation trainees did not have any training that was protected from service demands.[24] Almost two-thirds of trainees regularly worked beyond their rostered hours – this was a particular challenge for specialty trainees. The data indicated that Foundation and surgical trainees were particularly affected by the EWTD, highlighting the challenges of good rota design and the competing priorities of service and training.[24,29,33,34]

Additionally, the EWTD has led to reduced exposure to clinical activity and trainees are also less likely to experience continuity of patient care. The move away from an apprenticeship model to increased shift working has also led to a move away from the traditional 'firms' that have been central to the training of doctors in providing mentors and role models.[19] Concerns have also been raised about the increasing numbers of handovers and the decreasing amount of trainer–trainee time, with the risk of low supervision and training opportunities felt especially during the evenings or at night.

MEETING THE DEMANDS OF CHANGING POPULATIONS AND PATIENT EXPECTATIONS

Medical education is delivered within a constantly changing environment and needs to keep pace with both technological developments and rising patient expectations. Ageing populations and the increasing prevalence of long-term conditions and multiple pathologies will mean an increased need for high-quality end-of-life care. To meet these demands, reports have highlighted the need for Foundation doctors to be exposed to training across all care settings, including more community settings where much care of long-term conditions is now provided, along with more experience of working in multidisciplinary teams.[14,21] An evaluation of the Foundation Programme found that the distribution of placements by specialty does not reflect the current and future needs of the NHS, with placements mainly in adult medicine and surgery rather than primary care and the community.[21] The focus has largely been on acute illness but there are gaps in training for managing long-term conditions. Recent revisions to the Foundation curriculum seek to address this by strengthening the learning outcomes around management of long-term conditions acquired through community-based placements in specialties such as psychiatry, paediatrics, public health and general practice.[10] In addition, concerns have been raised that specialty training structures are not consistent with the need for more community care and that the structure of run-through training does not allow flexibility for trainees to transfer between specialties, making it difficult to adapt to changing healthcare needs and demand and to accommodate changing career choices of individual trainees.[14,19,35]

A further challenge of education and training relates to overseas-trained doctors, who now make up more than a third of registered doctors in the United Kingdom. The training system needs to provide better support and induction for these doctors to practise safely and to conform to ethical and professional standards in the United Kingdom.[14,36] The GMC is working with employers and professional organisations to develop a basic induction programme that all doctors would be required to complete before they start practising so that they are supported to treat patients safely.[14]

The challenge for NHS trusts is to deliver good education and training while maintaining services, meeting targets and implementing the working time directive. Ongoing reform has created further uncertainty about the future shape of healthcare and its ability to meet future demand with the limited resources available.

TIPS FOR MEDICAL STUDENTS AND JUNIOR DOCTORS

➤ It is never too early to start exploring various specialties for career options. Start by speaking to the careers adviser at your medical school.

➤ When you do your clinical placements, you could speak to Foundation doctors and specialty trainees already working in the specialties you have in mind. Then, try approaching educational or clinical supervisors working in the specialty to get further information.

➤ Attend local and/or national careers fairs to get additional information.

➤ Look up the relevant Royal College website to get further information, leaflets and other resources on specialty training.

➤ If you are not able to get first-hand experience of the specialty of choice, try to do a taster week using study leave during your Foundation training.

➤ Information on eligibility criteria, person specifications for specialties and competition ratios are available online for each specialty.

➤ Find out about the application forms, assessments used (numeric and verbal reasoning, situational judgement tests, etc.) and interview structure from relevant websites and by asking colleagues, and prepare your application and yourself well.

REFERENCES

1. Postgraduate Medical Education Training Board (PMETB). *Educating Tomorrow's Doctors: challenges for the future.* PMETB Briefing 002. London: PMETB; 2008.
2. Grant JR. Changing postgraduate medical education: a commentary from the United Kingdom. *Med J Aust.* 2007; **186**(7 Suppl.); S9–13.
3. Department of Health. *The NHS Plan: a plan for investment, a plan for reform.* London: The Stationery Office; 2000.
4. Donaldson L. *Unfinished Business: proposals for reform of the senior house officer grade.* London: Department of Health; 2002.
5. www.mmc.nhs.uk
6. General Medical Council (GMC). *The Trainee Doctor: foundation and specialty, including GP training.* London: GMC; 2011.
7. Department of Health. *Liberating the NHS: developing the healthcare workforce.* London: Department of Health; 2010.
8. General Medical Council (GMC). *Tomorrow's Doctors.* London: GMC; 2009.
9. Foundation Programme. *About the Programme.* Available at: www.foundation programme.nhs.uk/pages/home/about-the-foundation-programme (accessed 15 May 2012).
10. Foundation Programme. *The UK Foundation Programme Curriculum, 2012.* Available at: www.foundationprogramme.nhs.uk/pages/home/keydocs (accessed 6 June 2012).
11. UK Foundation Programme Office. *Foundation Programme Annual Report 2011: UK summary.* Report No. 3. Cardiff: UK Foundation Programme Office; 2011.
12. Working Group on Specialist Medical Training. *Hospital Doctors Training for the Future.* London; 1993.
13. NHS Executive. *A Guide to Specialist Registrar Training.* London: UK Departments of Health; 1998.
14. General Medical Council (GMC). *The State of Medical Education and Practice in the UK.* Manchester: GMC; 2011.
15. Department of Health Medical Education Training Programme Team. *Quick Guide to Recruitment to Medical Specialty Training in England 2012.* London: UK Department of Health 2012. Available at: www.mmc.nhs.uk/specialty_training/specialty_training_2012/recruitment_process/stage_1_-_getting_started/quick_guide__to_specialty_trai.aspx (accessed 5 June 2012).
16. Modernising Medical Careers. *Choosing Your Specialty.* London: MMC 2012. Available at: www.mmc.nhs.uk/specialty_training/specialty_training_2012/recruitment_process/stage_2_-_choosing_your_specia.aspx (accessed 31 May 2012).
17. General Medical Council. *Workplace Based Assessments.* London: GMC; 2010.
18. UK Health Departments. *The Gold Guide: a reference guide for postgraduate specialty training in the UK.* 4th ed. London: UK Health Departments; 2010.
19. Tooke J. *Aspiring to Excellence: findings and recommendations of the independent inquiry into Modernising Medical Careers.* London: MMC Inquiry; 2008.

20. Temple J. *Time for Training: a review of the impact of the European Working Time Directive on the quality of training.* London: Medical Education England; 2010.

21. Collins J. *Foundation for Excellence: an evaluation of the Foundation Programme.* London: Medical Education England; 2010.

22. E-Learning for Healthcare. *Foundation Programme.* Available at: www.e-lfh.org. uk/projects/foundation/index.html (accessed 25 June 2012).

23. General Medical Council (GMC). *National Training Surveys 2010: key findings.* Manchester: GMC; 2010.

24. General Medical Council (GMC). *National Training Survey 2011: key findings.* Manchester: GMC; 2011.

25. Illing J, Peile E, Morrison J, *et al. How Prepared are Medical Graduates to Begin Practice? A comparison of three diverse UK medical schools.* Final report for the GMC Education Committee. London: General Medical Council/Northern Deanery; 2008.

26. Dornan T, Ashcroft D, Heathfield H, *et al. An In-Depth Study Investigation into Causes of Prescribing Errors by Foundation Trainees in Relation to Their Medical Education.* Salford: Hope Hospital; 2009.

27. Goldacre MJ, Taylor K, Lambert TW. Views of junior doctors about whether their medical schools prepared them for work: questionnaire surveys. *BMC Med Educ.* 2010; **10**: 78.

28. Wakeling J, French F, Bagnall G, *et al.* Is Foundation training producing competent doctors? What do Foundation trainees, educational supervisors and nurses in Scotland have to say? *Scott Med J.* 2011; **56**(2): 87–93.

29. General Medical Council (GMC). *National Trainer Survey: key findings.* Manchester: GMC; 2011.

30. Academy of Medical Educators. *A Framework for the Professional Development of Postgraduate Medical Supervisors.* London: Academy of Medical Educators; 2010.

31. General Medical Council (GMC). *Recognising and Approving Trainers: a consultation.* London: GMC; 2012.

32. Moonesinghe SR, Lowery J, Shahi N, *et al.* Impact of reduction in working hours for doctors in training on postgraduate medical education and patients' outcomes: systematic review. *BMJ.* 2011; **342**: d1580.

33. Royal College of Surgeons of England. *Surgeons Call for Solution on Patient Safety and Future Training as Doctors Hours are Slashed.* London: Royal College of Surgeons of England; 23 January 2009. Available at: www.rcseng.ac.uk/ news/surgeons-call-for-solution-on-patient-safety-and-future-training-as-doctors-hours-are-slashed (accessed 15 May 2012).

34. Association of Surgeons in Training (ASiT). *Optimising Working Hours to Provide Quality in Training and Patient Safety.* London: ASiT; 2009. Available at: www.asit.org/assets/documents/ASiT_EWTD_Position_Statement.pdf (accessed 10 May 2012).

35. Spencer J. Generalism is dead. Long live generalism! In: Spencer J. *Monograph on the Foundation Programme.* Edinburgh: Association for the Study of Medical Education; 2007. pp. 17–20.

36. Illing J. *The Experiences of UK, EU and Non-EU Medical Graduates Making the Transition to the UK Workplace: full research report.* ESRC End of Award Report, RES-153-25-0097. Swindon: Economic and Social Research Council; 2009.

CHAPTER 4

The shifting sands of professional power

Alistair Leinster

INTRODUCTION

Traditionally, power within the healthcare sector has lain with doctors because of their expertise and arcane knowledge, which allowed them to define the nature of health and illness. They set the limits on what a patient could expect in terms of consultation and treatment, and they determined the standards by which they themselves would be judged. However, this power is being increasingly challenged by factors such as regulation of medical work, increased consumerism and lay involvement.[1] The nature of relationships with management within the complex organisations responsible for healthcare delivery remain poorly defined. Management, as referred to here, is the management team of a healthcare organisation – as opposed to the body of clinicians and healthcare professionals who directly deliver services. Within the UK acute healthcare sector this management team tends to comprise lower, middle and top managers who may or may not have a clinical background and whose roles focus solely on the management of services. Continuous change is now the norm within organisations,[2] and within healthcare this acts to further drive doctors and managers together. Despite this additional need to cooperate, a failure to understand each other's culture and viewpoint can lead to difficulties. This chapter sets out a framework based on a theoretical model that enables us to understand why these issues arise and how to better deal with them

Mintzberg's[3] description of organisational structure was selected as the basis for analysis, not only because of its relative simplicity and its consideration of sources of power within an organisation but also because it prompts the assessment of the management approach used in relation to specific organisational types. It sees five main organisational types ('simple structure', 'machine bureaucracy', 'professional bureaucracy', 'divisionalised form' and 'adhocracy'), and describes a range of characteristics and dynamics within each. The five organisational types are in turn defined and characterised within Mintzberg's[3] model by their organisational parts, mechanisms of coordination within the organisation and design parameters (e.g. job specialisation, performance control systems). Here, analysis focused on the professional bureaucracy as an organisational type, in relation to the healthcare sector.

POWER: MINTZBERG

Mintzberg's[3] description of a 'professional bureaucracy' as an organisational structure provides insight into the relationship between doctors and the organisations within which they work. As the UK National Health Service (NHS) is traditionally seen as an example of a professional bureaucracy,[4] Mintzberg's model[3] is particularly relevant in the United Kingdom, but the principles explored can be applied to the medical profession more broadly. The model is best viewed as a conceptual framework, helping us to comprehend organisational behaviour, rather than as a fixed typology.[5] It is within this spirit, acknowledging the risk of simplifying complex issues, that it is used here.

A number of the key characteristics of a professional bureaucracy[3] apply to doctors within healthcare organisations. These include jobs that are (1) highly specialised but minimally formalised, (2) require extensive training, and (3) with strong horizontal rather than vertical linkages. Clinicians work independently of administrative hierarchy and of each other, not only controlling their own work but also maintaining collective influence over administrative aspects of their organisation. The internal environment of professional bureaucracies is seen as complex but stable.[5] Complexity within a professional bureaucracy is seen by Mintzberg[5] to demand the use of skills and knowledge developed through prolonged training, while stability is seen as ensuring these skills become part of standard operating procedures with the organisation. This complex/stable environment has implications for the initiation and management of change and is often overlooked.

Mintzberg's wider model explores the interaction of different organisational components within each of the five main organisational structures. The key organisational component within the structure described as a professional bureaucracy is the 'operating core',[3] representing those who produce products or services. In the case of health services, a major component of this is the medical profession, in addition to nursing staff and other healthcare professionals. Much of the formal and informal power within a professional bureaucracy is held in this operating core rather than the 'strategic apex' (top general managers) or the 'middle line' (managers in direct line of authority between the operating core and the strategic apex).[5] Professionals' behaviour is predetermined by internalising the standardisation of skills[5] and particular values, which are inculcated or strengthened by professional training in healthcare.[6] The resultant lack of direct technical supervision that is observed in fully trained doctors[7] is another feature of a professional bureaucracy. Coordination within an organisation is achieved through the standardisation of skills, rather than of tasks or outputs. A reliance on internalised factors for control contrasts with external controls such as direct supervision or the standardisation of work processes that are seen within other organisational structures[5] and which are applied in many standard management approaches. Professional bureaucracies have been identified in a range of systems including accountancy firms, social work agencies, school systems and craft manufacturing[5] and are therefore not unique to healthcare. Allen[8] distinguishes doctors from some of these other groups by noting that unlike doctors, partners in these sectors will have to generate their own income, providing a different dynamic.

SOURCES OF POWER WITHIN A PROFESSIONAL BUREAUCRACY

A professional bureaucracy is characterised by the power of expertise.[3] Doctors share a large amount of specialised knowledge with one another[4] that has been inaccessible to others within healthcare organisations and to patients. This is reinforced by the practice of medicine requiring the acquisition of skills, gained through protracted and highly specialised training. The complexity of the medical work (the operating core within a professional bureaucracy) means that it cannot be easily formalised or its outputs be standardised through performance control systems or action planning.[5] As a result, the medical profession possesses a monopoly over the exercise of its work.[9] This perception is strengthened by professional self-regulation as the balance to clinical autonomy.[10] The professionals' power is legitimised through professional validation by a community of their peers.[11] In turn, this means that organisational configurations and structures with strong management or strategic control, where the work processes and outputs are standardised, are difficult to apply. While the application of Mintzberg's model focuses on power in relation to the organisations in which doctors work, similar themes of expertise and the impact of collegial mechanisms are seen to influence doctor–patient relationships.

Clinicians' acceptance of personal responsibility for patients and their sociolegal authority,[9] are important additional factors. They separate doctors from experts within other industries, giving them licence to influence the work of others from different disciplines. This leads to physicians intervening across an organisation, despite hierarchical and functional boundaries.[9] Again, this challenges the application of more generic approaches to management.

Interactions with healthcare management

Management within the NHS was originally expected to support the work of professionals by organising and providing resources.[12] Until the Griffiths Report in 1983,[13] which recommended the introduction of general management into the NHS, managers had little influence over doctors.[4] Although the need for healthcare management to move beyond a merely supportive role has been recognised, managers have yet to establish an agreed and accepted position in relation to doctors. Traditional management roles, approaches and power dynamics do not apply within the professional bureaucracies of health services. Organisational structures and approaches seen within other sectors, based on strong hierarchies, are ineffective. Attempts to reduce the power of the workforce or to control it through work standardisation or performance management are difficult, particularly in light of doctors' monopoly over their work and professional responsibility for their patients.

Within a healthcare organisation a clinician is relatively free of organisational hierarchy and unrestrained by subordination.[9] While, as will be discussed shortly, there are changes in relation to the power of clinicians within healthcare organisations, this can largely still be argued as being the case (particularly when compared with other staff groups within healthcare and in relation to other sectors). Healthcare managers are presented with a mandate and responsibility to manage resources and quality and deliver change, but given limited power to do so. While difficulties in working alongside the power base of clinicians are readily acknowledged, the sources of, or dynamics of that power are rarely explored explicitly or accounted for by managers. In addition, the lack of an agreed position between management and clinicians can lead to distracting and unhelpful plays for power and jurisdiction, with clinicians calling on their expertise and professional responsibility for their patients' care and managers calling on patient consumerism and the scarcity of resources, to legitimise their respective positions. In a stable environment the tacit concord arrived at within many organisations may work, but when significant change is required, latent tensions and conflict can soon arise and cause disruption.

The clinical director role was introduced within the United Kingdom with a view to engaging doctors in management through the creation of a doctor–manager role.[14] While this should enrich management decision-making and provide balance, tensions remain between managerial and professional structures. Thorne[10] conducted a case study to explore the role and impact of clinical directors on the medical profession. While she sees the clinical director as the nexus of clinical and managerial jurisdictions, her case study highlights the failure of this role to fully resolve the difficulties arising from the differing perspectives of management and clinicians. Within the case study, it appeared that managers failed to understand the collegial nature and dynamics of the medical profession. Managers expected clinical directors to use their position to control their colleagues, while their medical peers saw the role as having an obligation to defend the profession from management. The clinical directors' lack of managerial, organisational and contextual expertise disadvantaged them in decision-making and discussions, reducing their role to that of legitimising managers' corporate priorities.

Outcome measures and change in national policies in the United Kingdom

While state regulation supports the medical profession's monopoly over its work,[9] more recent developments in national policy within the United Kingdom are seen as contributing to a change of doctors' power. Decentralisation and increased local accountability at hospital trust level within the NHS has been linked to the increasing jurisdiction of chief executive officers, increasing their power in relation to doctors.[10] This was seen to give senior management increased power in relation to doctors, through mechanisms such as the selection and deployment of medical staff and the control of scarce resources. In addition, there is increased scrutiny of doctors through reporting and comparison of outcome measures as well as a drive to promote patient choice.

The white paper *Equity and Excellence: Liberating the NHS*[15] signalled a shift from monitoring processes within the NHS to that of outcomes. This was supported by *The NHS Outcomes Framework 2012/13*,[16] which established measures focused on the effectiveness of care, quality of patient experience and patient safety. In addition, a stated aim of the Patient Reported Outcome Measures programme[17] is to support the evaluation of clinical quality. Payment systems are also being adjusted to incentivise the reporting of quality within the NHS through the Commissioning for Quality and Innovation programme. This represents a drive to provide information on the quality of services as well as to support consumerism and patient choice. The opportunity for non-clinicians to compare the performance of doctors or their organisations, offered by increased information on quality of clinical services, contrasts with legitimisation and scrutiny of the medical profession being solely through validation by a community of peers.[11] Although the authority of doctors is not challenged directly, their right to claim it without justification is.

Relationship with patients

Doctors' professional relationship with patients, in itself characterised by the power of expertise, can be used as a negotiation tool in the interaction between the doctors and the managers within the professional bureaucracy. Recent developments in the formulation of the doctor–patient relationship itself present new challenges to the functioning of the bureaucracy. Whereas in the past, doctors saw themselves as the primary patient advocate mediating the patients' requirements to management, now the patients' and societal wishes are being mediated to the doctor through management. Examples of this dynamic include patient experience or consumerist based targets having potential to conflict with clinical prioritisation such as a 4-hour target for patients to receive treatment within emergency departments within the United Kingdom, and management initiated drives to develop patient-focused rather than professional-focused services.

Starr[11] reviews the nature of doctors' authority in relation to their patients. A doctor's professional authority is derived from their patients' dependence on their superior competence linking to the power of expertise, as discussed earlier. Authority is first defined as the possession of status or a quality that compels trust or obedience. Two forms are then distinguished – cultural and social. Cultural authority is the construction of reality through definitions of fact and value, while social authority is the ability to influence the actions of others. Both are seen as important in a doctor–patient interaction. The acceptance of a doctor's interpretation of signs and symptoms is the foundation of a doctor's cultural authority, which precedes any social authority. Within the context of a doctor–patient interaction it is social authority that persuades the patient to submit to treatment, follow advice or change their behaviour. In addition to the medical profession's power of expertise, its ability to solve practical problems is also important.[9] This requires not only the acceptance or rejection of diagnosis but also the acceptance of treatment. This separation of the acceptance of diagnosis, and of treatment options is an important distinction when considering changes in the power relationships between doctor and patient.

Power in relation to patients

The Royal College of Physicians Working Party report on medical professionalism in a changing world[18] describes the interaction between patient and doctor as a partnership, but one that is changing rapidly. However, the medical profession has been slow to adapt to changes in patient and societal expectations, with calls for a more active patient involvement in decision-making and the consultation process.

Doctor–patient interactions have traditionally been characterised by researchers as doctors exercising power over patients.[19] Despite an increased awareness of medical paternalism and communication skills training for doctors, the asymmetry in doctor–patient relationships persists. This indicates that the phenomenon has deeper roots than can be addressed simply through reform of the ways in which doctors talk to patients.[19] Patients are often in a vulnerable position when consulting a doctor, experiencing 'extraordinary moments of fear, anxiety and doubt'.[18] Patients are further disadvantaged by their ill-health, the unfamiliar environment and other stressors.[20] These factors reduce the power of patients, and disadvantage them in any interaction with the medical profession and contrast with those previously noted to underpin doctors' power.

Asymmetry within the doctor–patient relationship may be

inevitable and can, in some circumstances, be beneficial. Even Hippocrates stated, 'Some patients, though conscious that their condition is perilous, recover their health simply through their contentment with the goodness of the physician'[21]. However, dysfunctional asymmetry exists and is seen when patients have the ability to participate but are not allowed to. A range of negative manifestations of doctors' power include a patient not (1) taking charge of the consultation, (2) specifying their preferred outcome, (3) choosing the specialist to be referred to and (4) in the selection of medication. It can also be seen when the doctor asks more questions and interrupts the patient more than vice versa.[19] Further complaints include patients not feeling sufficiently involved in a consultation, not being able to ask questions or express their own ideas or concerns.[22]

Paternalism

Childress[23] defines paternalism as the failure of a doctor to acquiesce to a patient's wishes or choices, for the benefit of the patient. It is often justified on the basis of the principle of beneficence taking precedence over that of patient autonomy.[20] Alternatively, paternalism can be seen as a failure to fully account for a patient's views in interpreting a situation. Young[24] describes a hypothetical case of an active sportswoman who, against medical advice, requests analgesics to be given intravenously rather than by epidural, which would be more effective and lead to less discomfort, in order to avoid even a remote risk of being paralysed. Here, while the patient's competence is not questioned, her judgement differs from that of her doctor. This is not an example of conflict between patient autonomy and maleficence or beneficence as discussed by Duncan,[6] but, rather, of different interpretations of information, based on different sets of values.

Much of doctors' power has stemmed from a monopoly of knowledge about health and disease. This information is now available to the public, which both offers opportunities for engaging patients in their healthcare and poses difficult questions for the medical profession.[18] One issue raised in the Royal College of Physicians report in 2005 was the negotiation of differences in the interpretation of medical evidence between doctor and patient. This represents a challenging of doctors' cultural authority, with increasingly informed patients potentially testing a doctor's interpretation of signs and symptoms. Challenges to doctors' cultural authority (as a precursor to social authority, or the permission to give treatment or the acceptance of advice) need to be managed with care.

Shared decision-making

Increased acknowledgement of patient autonomy has led to calls for shared decision-making. Barratt[25] refers to shared decision-making as a paradigm shift in doctor–patient interactions. It is described as a move to empowering patients to actively participate in decision-making about their care. The current evaluation of shared decision-making relies on demonstrating its positive impact on health outcomes. This appears to suggest that the medical profession will consider shared decision-making only if it can be demonstrated to them that it improves health outcomes. A paradigm shift here would require that there is increased patient involvement in decision-making, providing it is does not result in a negative impact on health outcomes. Failure to embrace the notion of shared decision-making will have an adverse effect on the perception of the doctor as the primary patient advocate.

The established principles of informed consent, as captured in the NHS Patient's Charter,[26] provide a requirement for a clear explanation of proposed treatment which includes risks and alternatives prior to agreeing to treatment. This requires both the provision of appropriate levels of information, and the patient's right to choose. Earlier objections to this position by some practitioners were based on concerns about imparting information about procedures and risks, a wish to avoid causing anxiety or alarm, and problems of comprehension.[20] Earlier moves to a requirement for disclosure to patients to be based on what is considered by a reasonable healthcare practitioner under similar circumstances, were rejected in favour of a patient-centred approach. The principle of what a reasonable patient considered required information,[24] rather than what was reasonable to the doctor, was established. Framing discussions regarding shared decision-making in the context of those previously held in relation to informed consent, helps highlight the paradigm shift required in relation to shared decision-making and points to an ability of the profession to overcome complex issues in this area.

SUMMARY

The use of Mintzberg's model as a tool to aid reflection on the sources and nature of the power of the medical profession draws out a number of themes that have implications both for clinicians and managers of clinical services. Management of healthcare services needs to account for the power of expertise of its practitioners and their monopoly over the exercise of their work, difficulties standardising work and the professional responsibility doctors accept for their patients, which lead to a resistance to external control of the practitioner's activities. Despite the development of management within healthcare there is not yet a clear approach or model that addresses these points. Managers have to look beyond traditional management approaches used in other sectors that do not take account of the dynamics seen within healthcare. Clinicians will need to take an active role in facilitating a more positive interaction with managers and also ensure they develop sufficient knowledge and expertise to actively participate in management decision-making and discussions. The creation of the clinical director role may have helped to enrich decision-making and to partly bridge the gap between clinical and managerial perspectives, but it has failed to address many of the underlying dynamics. When considering this role, clinicians and managers need to be clear what is expected, and how it is intended to function within the organisation.

Within the United Kingdom, national policy is contributing to a changing position with regard to clinicians' power. Promotion of information to support patient choice and comparison of the effectiveness of individual clinicians is intended to empower patients. The development of national outcome measures widens the review of doctors' performance beyond a position of professional validation by a community of peers. This will continue to affect doctors' practice, as they are increasingly required to justify their authority by opening up to scrutiny, beyond that of self-regulation.

The doctor–patient relationship, previously determined by an unquestioned power of expertise, is changing on a number of fronts. Asymmetry in power relationships between doctors and patients has both functional and dysfunctional elements. Many of the dysfunctional elements are being challenged through increased calls for patient empowerment through mechanisms such as shared decision-making. Doctors need to develop positive ways to manage such elements through their practice, encouraging patient participation and better-informed patients without opening the door to constant challenge to their authority. If doctors fail to respond to patients' expectations, they risk losing their position as the primary patient advocate within the health system, as managers and health policymakers continue to engage with increasing societal demands.

REFERENCES

1. Allsop J, Mulchay L. *Regulating Medical Work*. Buckingham: Open University Press; 1996.
2. Jorgensen H, Owen L, Neus A. Stop improvising change management. *Strategy and Leadership*. 2009; 37(2): 38–44.
3. Mintzberg H. *The Structuring of Organisations*. Englewood Cliffs: Prentice Hall; 1979.
4. Dickinson H, Ham C. *Engaging Doctors in Leadership: review of the literature*. Birmingham: University of Birmingham; 2008.
5. Mintzberg H. Structure in 5's: a synthesis of the research on organization design. *Manage Sci*. 1980; 26(3): 322–41.
6. Duncan P. *Critical Perspectives on Health*. Basingstoke: Palgrave MacMillan; 2007.
7. Unger J, Macq J, Bredo F, *et al*. Through Mintzberg's glasses: a fresh look at the organization of ministries of health. *Bull World Health Organ*. 2000; 78(8): 1005–13.
8. Allen D. Doctors in management or the revenge of the conquered: the role of management development for doctors. *J Manag Med*. 1995; 9(4): 44–50.
9. Freidson E. *Profession of Medicine: a study of the sociology of applied knowledge*. Chicago, IL: University of Chicago Press; 1988.
10. Thorne ML. Colonizing the new world of NHS management: the shifting power of professionals. *Health Serv Manage Res*. 2002; 15(1): 14–26.
11. Starr P. *The Social Transformation of American Medicine*. New York, NY: Basic Books; 1982.
12. Harrison S. *Managing the National Health Service: shifting the frontier?* London: Chapman & Hall; 1988.
13. Department of Health and Social Security. *NHS Management Inquiry Report* (Griffiths Report). London: HMSO; 1983.
14. McKee L, Marnoch G, Dinnie N. Medical managers: puppetmasters or puppets? Sources of power and influence in clinical directorates. In: Mark A, Dopson S, editors. *Organisational Behaviour in Health Care: the research agenda*. Basingstoke: Macmillan Press; 1999. pp. 89–116.
15. Department of Health. *Equity and Excellence: liberating the NHS*. London: The Stationery Office; 2010.
16. Department of Health. *The NHS Outcomes Framework 2012/13*. London: The Stationery Office; 2011.
17. Department of Health. *Patient Reported Outcome Measures (PROMs) in England: a methodology for identifying outliers*. London: The Stationery Office; 2012.
18. Royal College of Physicians (RCP). *Doctors in Society: medical professionalism in a changing world*. Report of a Working Party of the Royal College of Physicians of London. London: RCP; 2005.
19. Pilnick R, Dingwall R. On the remarkable persistence of asymmetry in doctor/patient interaction: a critical review. *Soc Sci Med*. 2011; 72(8): 1374–82.
20. Singleton J, McLaren S. *Ethical Foundations of Health Care: responsibilities in decision making*. London: Mosby; 1995.

21. Hippocrates. *Precepts VI* (date uncertain). English translation available at http://perseus.uchicago.edu/perseus-cgi/citequery3.pl?dbname=GreekTexts &query=Hipp.%20Praec.%208&getid=1 (accessed 30 January 2013).

22. Maguire P. Communication skills and patient care. In: Steptoe A, Mathews A, editors. *Health Care and Human Behaviour*. London: Academic Press; 1984. pp. 153–73.

23. Childress JF. *Who Should Decide? Paternalism in health care*. Oxford: Oxford University Press; 1982.

24. Young R. Informed consent and patient autonomy. In: Kuhse H, Singer P, editors. *A Companion to Bioethics*. 2nd ed. Oxford: Wiley-Blackwell; 2012. pp. 530–40.

25. Barratt A. Evidence based medicine and shared decision making: the challenge of getting both evidence and preferences into health care. *Patient Educ Couns*. 2008; **73**(3): 407–12.

26. Department of Health. *The Patient's Charter: raising the standards*. London: The Stationery Office; 1992.

CHAPTER 5

Doctors in management

Penny Cavenagh and Bernard Brett

INTRODUCTION

Doctors' roles in the twenty-first century are being dramatically redefined across many dimensions,[1] and one that has been bubbling away for more than 25 years is their involvement in the management of their employing organisations and healthcare systems. This chapter will explore the reasons and ways in which doctors are becoming involved in increasing numbers and in ever more sophisticated roles in management within the National Health Service (NHS), despite a long period of reluctance to do so.

THE EVOLUTION OF DOCTORS AS CLINICAL MANAGERS

Doctors remained free from any significant involvement in management for the first 40 years of the NHS, almost enjoying self-employed status. They had the freedom and autonomy to decide how to treat their patients, while feeling confident that their decisions would be implemented effectively. The medical profession has had a strong focus on knowledge, pattern recognition (reaching a diagnosis when confronted with a familiar constellation of symptoms) and procedural skills with less focus on reliable delivery of care. Even for well-established aspects of patient management (such as undertaking a particular type of assessment or the delivery of a specific medication), delivery rarely achieves 90% reliability, which means that patient safety and patient outcomes can be adversely affected. An example of this is the recent drive to improve the rate of venous thromboembolism risk assessments within hospitals. With much work and leadership driven from a national, regional and local level and aligned financial incentives, it has taken many months to achieve levels above 90% – this improvement has only been delivered with clinical involvement in leading and managing change.

THE CONCEPT OF CLINICAL FREEDOM

This concept of 'clinical freedom' has been extremely important to the medical profession, although its meaning has been differentially interpreted by doctors. For some it has been the desire to deliver the best possible care to patients, whereas others have viewed it as freedom and autonomy from management or interference from other members of the medical profession.[2] This freedom to determine what is in the best interests of the patient based on individual clinicians' knowledge, experience and beliefs has contributed to the significant local, regional and national variation in practice and care delivery. Clinical needs of individual patients have thus historically provided the focus for doctors' decision-making,[3] and by making decisions for patient care management doctors have always contributed in some way to the 'management process'.[3] However, they have often had no 'corporate accountability' for resources or for managing other staff.[4]

DOCTORS' COVERT ROLE IN MANAGEMENT

Doctors have, however, always had a responsibility for people management. As doctors have moved up through the medical hierarchy, they have had a responsibility for the performance, as well as the training, of those reporting to them. This responsibility has not been as well articulated with clear accountability as it is in other professions. Additionally, doctors have not seen this as 'management'; rather, this area has been viewed as 'training'. In addition, general practice partners have throughout the history of the NHS had a managerial role in the responsibility in the running of their general practices, including the management of non-medical staff, yet in general they would not wish to be seen as managers but as clinicians.

THE DEVELOPMENT AND TRAINING OF MEDICAL MANAGERS

Despite the increasing need for management skills, doctors have rarely been trained to improve their management and leadership capability in a significant way. Over recent years doctors in training would usually be expected to have undertaken a management course before consultant appointment. However, this would likely be a desirable rather than essential component of the person specification for posts and a course for a day or two would usually be considered sufficient during the appointment process.

THE DRIVERS FOR INCREASING MEDICAL INVOLVEMENT IN MANAGEMENT

The challenges the NHS face today are as great, if not even greater, than ever before. Advances in medical technology, the increasing needs of an ageing population, new drugs and treatment, and rising expectations of better care are making excessive demands on and outstripping available NHS resources. Critical choices are being made, weighing up the costs and benefits of all aspects of NHS provision. Every clinical decision made by doctors draws upon a hospital's resources[5] and it therefore has seemed only logical to involve doctors in the management of the increasingly scarce resources of the NHS. Successive governments, particularly since the mid-1970s, have been more and more determined to involve doctors in management with only limited success. One such attempt (emerging from the Griffiths Report[6]) involved the introduction of general managers in the place of teams charged with decision-making. However, this attempt failed to improve efficiency by involving doctors in management.[4] The purpose of the Griffiths strategy was to appoint members of the medical profession to general management posts in the United Kingdom. However, only 9.5% of these posts were taken up by doctors.[7]

The introduction of clinical directorates and the appointment of clinical directors and medical directors as a result of the 1991 reorganisation[8] of the NHS was the first real phase of medical management in NHS trusts. Similarly, the establishment of general practitioner (GP) fundholding and practice-based commissioning heralded the first involvement of doctors in the management of resources in primary care. The directorate model involved the creation of managerial subunits or specialisms,[9] which were established as a method of ensuring that responsibility and power was devolved to clinicians.[10] The key purpose was, therefore, to unify rather than separate the practice of management and medicine in NHS trusts. This model of medical management with clinician leads, clinical directors and or divisional directors is now embedded in NHS trust structures.[11] There is no single best model for clinical directorates, and roles, relationships and responsibilities vary between trusts. The determination of the management structure most appropriate for the organisation is the responsibility of the chief executive.[12]

There are many issues for doctors inherent in the clinical director role, including lack of time,[12] but one of the key problems is the perception that clinical directors have of themselves as clinicians first and managers second. This has led to problems of 'role incompatibility' and 'role conflict', owing to the frequent clash of clinical and management values.[9] The concept of professional identity largely underpins the problem of role incompatibility. A study of clinical directors[4] highlighted the importance of clinical directors retaining their *clinical* professional identity. The clinical directors in this study maintained allegiance primarily with their medical colleagues, focusing on their clinical work in order to avoid professional isolation. Indeed, fear of professional alienation from their colleagues has been strong motivation to avoid involvement in management.[12-14] Numerous studies have evidenced the reluctance of doctors to be involved in management and the reasons why.[13,15] Many doctors have found it difficult to combine clinical and management responsibilities, and some felt that they had been bullied into taking on management roles or were fearful of being managed.

However, despite this reticence some doctors are keen to take on management roles both because of their commitment to quality patient care and because of a desire to contribute and add value to their organisation in a broader role. They also believe that they can effect change and perhaps do a better job than other medical colleagues.[16]

THE REDEFINING OF DOCTORS' ROLES IN MODERN HEALTHCARE

The financial- and market-oriented climate of hospitals in all 'industrialised economies' has changed to the extent that in the twenty-first century, doctors and managers can no longer afford not to collaborate and work together. To not do so could pose a threat to the survival of hospitals.[17] A recent study on physicians in two hospitals in Germany suggested that a successful hospital career is now partly dependent on some degree of focus on management.[17]

The emphasis on doctors acquiring clinical leadership and management skills is evidenced by the introduction of the Medical Leadership Competency Framework.[1] This framework has been co-developed by the Academy of Medical Royal Colleges and the NHS Institute for Innovation and Improvement, and it defines those leadership competencies necessary for doctors to be successful and effective in their careers.[1] Indeed, the requirement for doctors today to demonstrate competence in leadership and management calls into question the whole concept of what it is to be 'professional'[1] in medicine.

The ethos of professionalism traditionally socialised into medical students could be seen to be at odds with a possible reframing of what it may mean to be professional for a doctor in the twenty-first century. Indeed the emerging redefinition of professionalism appears to be in response to economic challenges and the need to exercise the concept of opportunity cost in the increasingly austere financial climate of the NHS.

Historically the success of the professions has been built upon service to an individual and the hallmark of professionalism is the relationship between the professional and client.[18] The success of medicine is attributed to the 'powerful' relationship between doctor and patient and the belief and trust that the doctor will work and make decisions in their 'best interest'.[19] A further key aspect of professionalism is the focus on the 'technical' rather than 'non-technical' basis of the role.[20] As applied to the medical profession, this could be interpreted as clinical rather than non-clinical/managerial facets of the role.

DOCTORS' PROFESSIONAL IDENTITY

Doctors' professional identity is predicated on this trusted relationship with their patients, dispensing specialist and expert medical knowledge on an individual basis. Involvement in management and the reframing of what it means to be professional necessitates the consideration by doctors of aggregate health needs across a defined population rather than individual health needs. This invariably will involve some degree of choice in terms of service provision and delivery. It may involve doctors compromising in terms of 'best interest' in individual patient care and to challenge the foundation of their core beliefs and professional identity. The emphasis on 'generic' and 'non-technical' use of skills may again threaten professional identity. The very recent introduction of clinical commissioning groups is necessitating GPs to also make strategic decisions about resource allocation and health needs of the total population in the community they represent. This is at odds with their traditional professional role as patient advocates for each individual.

Harvey-Jones[21] in 1996 was keen to point out that the medical and legal professions could do far more with their professional skills if they embraced management roles. Fifteen years on, medical professionals have become more involved in key roles in the management of NHS resources, and this is increasing further. Doctors today expect to be involved, albeit to varying degrees, in this type of management activity whether they are working in primary or secondary care. Perhaps involvement in management will become part of a doctor's professional identity rather than at odds with it, particularly as they progress through their careers. The more pervasive this shift becomes the more it may become entrenched in the definition of professionalism. What it means to be professional perhaps needs to be reframed to include a focus not only on the individual but also on aggregate need, a focus not only on the 'technical' but also on the 'non' technical, and a focus not only on clinical knowledge and skills but also on effective delivery of care.

THE INCREASING NEED FOR CLINICAL INVOLVEMENT IN NATIONAL HEALTH SERVICE MANAGEMENT

In the NHS today there is an increasing need for clinical input from all healthcare professionals (nurses, therapists, etc.), especially medical (doctors), into a range of management activities and an increasing need for management and leadership skills among doctors at all levels. This has been created by many factors including: changes in care delivery such as Hospital at Night (where junior doctors' management and leadership skills are a necessity for an efficient, safe service); the Next Stage review, which was commissioned by the last Labour government to update the NHS Plan and was led by Lord Darzi (which has led to an increased focus on quality in terms of safety, effectiveness and experience requiring clinical involvement in designing and delivering change); the introduction of the Commissioning for Quality and Innovation (CQUIN) programme; the introduction of quality accounts (giving a comprehensive overview of each trust's quality performance on an annual basis); Quality Outcomes Framework in primary care (incentive payments for the achievement of specified quality targets); and best practice tariff (enhanced payment for delivering defined key aspects of care for each patient with a particular condition rather than payment based purely on the number of patients treated) – all of which require clinical involvement in the commissioning and delivery of services.

Taking just one example of these new factors, the CQUIN programme was introduced through the NHS commissioning framework in 2009, initially accounting for 1% of NHS trusts' budgets and now accounting for 2.5%. CQUINs incentivise trusts to deliver quality improvements and innovations in care. They need significant clinical input to determine appropriate themes, goals and key performance indicators that are relevant in a local healthcare system and subsequently to determine whether or not milestones and performance indicators have been achieved. Significant clinical input is also required to ensure that organisations deliver against these targets.

In addition to these examples, as already discussed, the biggest driver increasing the need for medical leadership and management is the current financial squeeze on NHS resources on a background of increasing demand for those resources generated through demography, medical advances and public expectation. This need to maintain or improve quality (in terms of measureable outcomes for patients), and meet patient expectations (including a good experience of care) while reducing costs requires significant changes in the way patients are treated. These changes to patient pathways (the sequence of all relevant episodes of care and communication that relate to a single presentation or new condition) can only be delivered with significant clinical involvement and leadership. The establishment of clinical commissioning groups by the current coalition government is an attempt to ensure increased clinical involvement in the management of the health service and has created significant demand for clinical leadership and management within the structure of the NHS.

The NHS strives to develop and deliver Quality, Innovation, Productivity and Prevention plans. These are made up of a series of projects, where streamlined innovative, efficient healthcare pathways deliver quality improvement while driving down costs. Simple examples of how these two aims can be aligned include the reduction in complications and more early senior assessment for patients attending hospital as an emergency. Reducing complications such as healthcare associated infections, pressure ulcer or falls can reduce length of stay in hospital and treatment costs. Earlier senior clinician involvement and diagnostics in emergency cases can lead to the timelier implementation of appropriate patient management plans, reducing avoidable admissions and the length of stay for those who are admitted.

In order to achieve this challenging agenda it is necessary to streamline clinical pathways and processes, with increased standardisation and reduced variation. This can only be achieved with not just clinical input but also clinical leadership and engagement. Whole teams need to be encouraged, persuaded or occasionally performance managed to deliver change. A variety of methodologies (such as lean, described shortly) have been used to help clinicians and other managers deliver high-quality efficient care. The understanding and application of these methodologies are prime examples of the need for non-clinical skills among doctors to enable them to lead, input or at least engage with change processes in the modern NHS.

The NHS, and indeed healthcare worldwide, is increasingly trying to learn from other industries.[22] There is drive within the NHS to incorporate lean methodology or one of its variants into healthcare. One of the most heralded non-healthcare examples of a lean approach is the Toyota production system and it is hoped that if the NHS were to use a similar approach it could simultaneously improve quality, morale and productivity. There are many elements to the approach used in the Toyota production system, including seeing all work as an end-to-end process and determining whether each step is adding value or not. Non-value-added or wasteful steps are then eliminated – typically such steps are said to outnumber value-added steps in a ratio 9:1. Another key element of the Toyota approach is creating order and cleanliness or the improvement of workplace layout and organisation. This will then minimise staff movement and reduce excessive stock, resulting in efficiency and cost-effectiveness.[22] Medical staff have rarely been trained in such methodology but this may well have a greater impact on patient outcomes than much of the training focusing on increasing knowledge and procedural skills. A far greater number of adverse incidents occur as a result of a failure to follow a well-recognised guideline or pathway rather than as a result of a lack of knowledge or procedural skills.

One of the most cited examples of cost-effective high-quality healthcare provision and delivery is Kaiser Permanente, a not-for-profit healthcare insurer based in North America. This organisation's leadership is very heavily clinically based and has demonstrated high-quality health outcomes with low bed utilisation and low cost.[23,24] They have focused on quality outcomes and prevention. They also focus on continuous service improvement, with dedicated teams to help deliver this. It is one of the cheapest US healthcare providers, yet its medical results are also impressive; by many clinical measurements it is the best performing healthcare provider in the regions in which it operates.[25]

Several NHS healthcare systems have tried to emulate elements of the Kaiser approach including three pilot sites in Birmingham and Solihul, Northumbria, and Torbay.[26] Torbay in particular has managed to significantly reduce its use of acute hospital beds.[27] There are many elements to the Kaiser approach including integration of care, a focus on chronic care and population management, with self-management also being a key component. A much higher proportion of doctors take on leadership roles with doctors playing a key role in decision-making and driving clinically focussed change. A significant investment is made on leadership development. Kaiser also has a strong focus on service improvement and utilising lean type methodologies.

It is unlikely that higher-quality, more streamlined care alone will enable healthcare systems to meet the challenge of increasing demand and expectations with significantly constrained financial funding. Most, if not all, commissioning organisations are either exploring or already introducing thresholds (cut-off levels that determine whether or not an individual is eligible for a particular procedure through the NHS) for some types of treatment, usually surgical operations, to reduce clinical activity and therefore costs. Clinical involvement is vital to ensure that thresholds are set based on relevant clinical factors and that their impact on the quality of care is minimised.

CONCLUDING REMARKS

The medical management structures and therefore opportunities in many organisations have changed considerably over recent years. The traditional model of a medical director and several clinical directors in secondary and tertiary care units is changing. Increasingly it is recognised that the senior medical management portfolio has grown such that many organisations have one or more deputy medical directors or associate medical directors. Below this management layer there are often divisional directors with broader portfolios than clinical directors. Similarly, clinical commissioning organisations in every region need primary care physicians to operate at board level and at the commissioning level. This requires a big increase in the number of GPs needed for management roles. Private care and third sector organisations are providing other significant management opportunities for doctors that are likely to increase further with policy changes such as the approach to any willing provider.

Doctors' roles are being redefined and one of the biggest changes is their involvement in management and leadership at all levels and in all organisations within the NHS. The need for such changes has been driven by many factors, the most significant of which is a challenging financial environment with increased demand for healthcare. Increasingly the need to focus on aggregate health benefits more than individual health benefits with an increased need to enhance and use non-clinical skills is changing what it means to be a medical professional.

RECOMMENDATIONS

There is steadily increasing need for doctors at all levels to take on managerial roles and leadership roles.

➤ This need should be supported through a greater emphasis in developing appropriate skills at both undergraduate and postgraduate level.

➤ Individual doctors need to recognise the opportunities and challenges of the changing environment and ensure that they gain appropriate levels of training and experience in management and leadership.

➤ The medical profession needs to recognise the importance of medical leadership in ensuring that we can deliver high-quality healthcare in a challenging financial and demographic environment with the real terms reduction in funding and increasing demand.

REFERENCES

1. Clark J, Armit K. Attainment of competency in management and leadership: no longer an optional extra for doctors. *Clin Govern Int J.* 2009; 13(1): 35–42.
2. Saxton H. Personal perspectives. In: Burrows M, Dyson R, Jackson P, *et al.*, editors. *Management for Hospital Doctors.* Oxford: Butterworth-Heinemann; 1994.
3. Marnoch G. *Doctors and Management in the National Health Service.* Buckingham: Open University Press: 1996.
4. Thorne ML. Being a clinical director: first among equals or just a go-between? *Health Serv Manage Res.* 1997; 10(4): 205–15.
5. Simpson J. Doctors as managers: juniors and seniors. *Br J Hosp Med.* 1995; 54(4): 173–4.
6. Department of Health and Social Security (DHSS). *NHS Management Enquiry.* Griffiths Report DA (83)38. London: HMSO; 1983.
7. Alleway L. No rush of new blood into the NHS. *Health Soc Serv J.* 1985; 95(4965); 1120–1.
8. Department of Health and Social Security (DHSS). *Working for Patients.* London: HMSO; 1989.
9. Willcocks S. The clinical director in the NHS utilising a role-theory perspective. *J Manage Med.* 1994; 8(5): 68–75.
10. Mark A. Where are the medical managers? *J Manage Med.* 1991; 54(4): 6–12.
11. Palmer R, Raynor H, Way D. Multisource feedback: 360° degree assessment of professional skills of clinical directors. *Health Serv Manage Res.* 2007; 20(3): 183–8.

12. Buchanan D, Jordan S, Preston D, *et al.* Doctors in the process: the engagement of clinical directors in hospital management. *J Manage Med.* 1997; **11**(3): 132–56.

13. Dopson S. Management: the one disease consultants did not think existed. *J Manage Med.* 1994; **18**(5): 25–36.

14. Riordan J, Simpson J. Getting started as a medical manager. *BMJ.* 1994; **309**(10): 1563–5.

15. Simpson J, Scott T. *Leading Clinical Services: the evolving role of the clinical director. Bamm & Cranfield School of Management Survey.* Cheadle, Cheshire: British Association of Medical Managers; 1997.

16. Cavenagh P. Buggins' turn or Buggins' choice: a sequel. *Clin Manage.* 2000; **9**(3): 146–59.

17. Vera A, Hucke D. Managerial orientation and career success of physicians in hospitals. *J Health Organ Manag.* 2009; **23**(1): 70–84.

18. Schon DA. *The Reflective Practitioner: how professionals think in action.* New York, NY: Basic Books; 1983.

19. Moore GT. Doctors as managers: frustrating tensions. In: Costain D, editor. *The Future of Acute Services: doctors as managers.* London: King's Fund Centre; 1990.

20. Parsons T. *The Social System.* London: Routledge & Kegan Paul; 1951.

21. Harvey-Jones, Sir J. Cited in: Coles M. Managing for professionals. *Sunday Times.* 1996; 17 November.

22. Fillingham D. Can lean save lives? *Leadersh Health Serv (Bradf Engl).* 2007; **20**(4): 231–41.

23. Ham C, York N, Sutch S, *et al.* Hospital bed utilisation in the NHS, Kaiser Permanente, and the US Medicare programme: analysis of routine data. *BMJ.* 2003; **327**(7426): 1257–62.

24. Feachem RGA, Sekhri N, White KL. Getting more for their dollar: a comparison of the NHS with California's Kaiser Permanente. *BMJ.* 2002; **324**: 135–43.

25. Controlling health-care costs: another American way. *The Economist.* 2010; April 29.

26. Ham C. *Working Together for Health: achievements and challenges in the Kaiser NHS Beacon sites programme.* Policy paper 6. Birmingham: Health Service Management Centre, University of Birmingham; 2010.

27. Davies P. A glimpse of the future of healthcare at the seaside. *BMJ.* 2011; **342**: d1917.

CHAPTER 6

Accountability, performance and targets

Richard Young and Krishna Sethia

In his 1937 book *The Citadel*,[1] AJ Cronin describes the career of a young country doctor who is first seduced but later horrified by medical practice in London. His attempt to expose poor practice results in a vicious reaction from the medical establishment that results in him being brought before the General Medical Council. In a subsequent interview Cronin said, 'I have written in *The Citadel* all I feel about the medical profession, its injustices, its hide-bound unscientific stubbornness, its humbug . . . The horrors and inequities detailed in the story I have personally witnessed. This is not an attack against individuals, but against a system.'[2] *The Citadel* is often said to be one of the drivers that resulted in the formation of the National Health Service (NHS) some 11 years later. It can also be viewed as a portrayal of the regulatory framework in place at the time – more concerned with protecting the reputation and interests of the medical profession than with holding doctors to account.

This chapter outlines the nature and scope of the changes occurring in the relationship between the medical profession and the direct and indirect users of the profession – namely, patients and government/providers, respectively. It documents the introduction of ideas of performance management and monitoring for doctors, and the tools that have been used to achieve this. It is written from a UK perspective and as such is influenced heavily by the development of the NHS, which has dominated the landscape of UK healthcare from the middle of the twentieth century. However, most if not all of the factors described in relation to doctors' accountability also apply in societies across the Western world, regardless of the type of health-care system in place. While the NHS was designed for the benefit of patients, its highly visible role as a cornerstone of the welfare state has meant that in its 64 years politicians have constantly sought to use it to gain advantage. It was only when they realised that pressures on the whole health system always continue to increase that they began to attempt to involve clinicians in its management. However, even with recent governments emphasising the importance of clinical leadership, they have found it impossible to relinquish control and at times remain guilty of micromanagement of the system.

An example of this is the way in which the Labour government of the early 2000s introduced a range of mandatory waiting list targets for acute hospitals. These were attached to stringent penalties should the targets be breached; while they were a powerful tool to improve access targets for individual patients, they were rarely underpinned by sound clinical imperatives and so struggled to engage clinical staff. Without this engagement it was, and must remain, very difficult to manage performance of clinicians.

Unfortunately, even for those clinicians who are keen to devote the necessary time and energy, the current structure of the NHS provides significant obstacles to effective performance management. Perhaps most significant is the lack of agreement about what constitutes good performance. Most clinicians think that good performance should be defined according to clinical outcomes (e.g. survival rates, incidence of complications after surgery). However, hospital managers, usually driven by political imperatives, may be as keen to ensure compliance with waiting time targets or control of the healthcare spend. In his 2008 report *High Quality Care for All*,[3] Lord Darzi described good-quality care as being determined by a combination of factors: clinical outcomes, patient safety, patient experience, access, equality and efficiency. The challenge remains how to achieve a sensible balance between these aspirations and not just those dictated by the political flavour of the day.

A second difficulty in implementing performance management is the lack of relevant and complete data, especially for clinical outcomes. The new lists of NHS performance indicators (e.g. cancer referral waiting times, cancelled operations) are a useful attempt to provide a basis for comparing results from different hospitals, but even they do not include full assessment of risk factors, which may affect outcomes. Organisations such as Dr Foster Intelligence supply data on individual performance but with very broad confidence limits and no long-term survival data. Although some national registers (e.g. cardiothoracic surgery) are sufficiently mature to allow comparisons, in general there are few reliable systems that allow useful comparison of individual clinical outcomes.

Measuring the performance of trainee doctors in the NHS has become even more difficult. Implementation of the European Working Time regulations and the New Deal for junior doctors has resulted in those doctors having to work in shift systems rather than being continuously available. This has resulted in the breakdown of the 'firm' structure (the 'firm' was the traditional structure for medical teams in the UK hospital sector, involving usually one consultant, at least one middle-grade specialist trainee, and at least one entry-grade trainee) and potential lack of accountability. During a single admission a patient may be looked after by several junior doctors, some of whom may be completely unknown to the consultant in charge of the case – the consultant is therefore unlikely to be aware of any errors or problems arising as a result of a junior doctor's management of that patient. While it is true that there have been improvements in supervision and training of junior doctors, this in itself puts demands on consultant time that have increased dramatically and are at risk of becoming unaffordable to the service.

Allowing for these difficulties, it remains essential that clinicians should be involved in managing performance. A demonstration of the potential benefit of this approach is seen in the Kaiser Permanente Group in the United States, where groups of doctors determine the nature and extent of the service to be provided to patients. At Kaiser, clinicians both receive regular feedback on a series of parameters accepted to be of clinical importance and also use committees of clinicians to monitor and if necessary police clinical activities of the group. The challenge for the NHS remains how to introduce this clinical leadership most effectively.

Medical involvement with management, and responsibility for resource utilisation, began in earnest with general practitioner (GP) fundholding. This attempted to apply the principles of Adam Smith, the eighteenth-century philosopher and exponent of the principles of free markets, to the field of a state-funded health economy. Although it was originally ideologically driven, it soon became apparent that this was a powerful political tool. It set doctors up in competition with one another, made transparent differences in quality and efficiency of care, and allowed politicians to shrug off responsibility for rationing of resources, which by the mid-1990s had become a major issue in the NHS. Fundholding did appear to offer a number of benefits. First was the fact that for the first time the health system was required to calculate the cost of procedures, drugs and different forms of care. Second, by empowering GPs to negotiate over the costs of treatment in secondary care, they were able to drive prices down. Third, it put clinicians in a position of influence regarding purchasing priorities and decisions. However, fundholding also had a number of significant disadvantages. By forcing secondary care and other providers to compete with one another, sometimes for their very survival, some procedures and care were carried out at less than cost price, which was clearly not sustainable in the long term. Many of the savings that were made from fundholding were marginal, based on the 'lowest hanging fruit' principle (that is, easy to procure but with little significance) while other areas where more major cost savings could have been made were ignored. Finally, the system was incentivised by allowing GPs to determine to a large extent how the cost savings would be utilised. In most cases, savings were ploughed back into the wider healthcare economy, but there were instances of significant amounts of money benefiting the practices directly in the form of improved premises or equipment purchases in primary care. While this may not have been a probity issue, there is no doubt that this sort of activity did not give fundholding a good name.

The principle that doctors need to take an interest in resource allocation has outlived fundholding and, indeed has now become one of the tenets of the General Medical Council's *Good Medical Practice*.[4] Hospitals are now engaged in service line reporting, which in effect informs them of the cost of individual procedures for individual patients. While feedback of this information to clinical directorates or individual consultants remains variable, it is undoubtedly a tool that has the potential to change practice. On a larger scale, primary care commissioning groups, created by the Health and Social Care Act 2012 and charged with identifying the best way to provide care, will need to be constantly aware of potential financial savings that may be achieved, either by effective procurement or by alternative service provision – for example, investing in admission avoidance initiatives rather than allowing more expensive hospital admissions.

This last example illustrates a further difficulty – the fact that incentives in the NHS are poorly aligned to the objectives of the service. Although clinical commissioning now (partly) resides with GPs, GPs remain independent businesses whose attempts to save resource may add pressure on other parts of the system. Similarly, it may be in the interest of hospital trusts to manage patients without considering the additional pressure that may ensue for primary care. Until there is proper (including financial) integration of all parts of the NHS, it is difficult to see how efficiency can be maximised.

A potential advantage of commissioning is that it can be used to ensure that services attain a predefined standard. An example of how this is already being used in the NHS is the withholding of a proportion of a hospital's income unless it achieves pre-agreed quality targets, so-called Commissioning for Quality and Innovation. This proportion is now 4% of a hospital's budget and may increase with time. Unfortunately, this is now combined with the threat of draconian penalties for hospitals failing to achieve certain national quality targets. This approach may be misguided, as incentives and/or threats do not necessarily improve healthcare performance.[5] Commissioning also encourages efficiency by demanding that patients are managed in standard ways, the so-called best care pathways.

The increasing need for clinicians to be engaged in and accountable for decisions about the use of resources in the healthcare system has been a driver for the advance of evidence-based medicine/practice (EBM) in the United Kingdom. While it is undoubtedly true that the more widespread adoption of EBM ensures that patients receive treatments that are effective and, in particular, that patients do not receive treatments that are of limited benefit or are even positively harmful, it is also true that these changes have had a fundamental effect on the nature of the doctor–patient relationship. Patients are very aware that doctors are now engaged in rationing decisions, and while they may be comfortable with this and accept it on a population level, for the individual in a consultation with a doctor the question frequently arises, 'is it because this is too expensive, Dr?'

While successive administrations have attempted to tackle the perceived inefficiencies of secondary care since at least 1990, performance targets in primary care are a relatively recent phenomenon. The new GP contract of 2004 changed the landscape of primary care overnight. It included a system of quality payments called the Quality and Outcomes Framework (QuOF). For example, GPs were paid a sum, per patient, for ensuring that repeat medication was subject to an annual review, or for achieving target blood pressures in the majority of their hypertensive patients. Significantly, the new contractual arrangements involved removing a large proportion of funding from the basic practice allowance, and this could only be earned back by succeeding within the QuOF; GPs, therefore, had very little option other than to participate. A discipline that had always prided itself as being the most patient centred in medicine found itself with the challenge of trying to meet a whole range of performance targets related to patient care. While many of these targets had a strong evidence basis and a robust rationale for universal application (e.g. prescribing of statins to patients with established ischaemic heart disease), others have been more contentious (e.g. discussion of long-acting reversible contraception with *all* patients presenting for family planning advice). Many general practitioners resented such interference with clinical freedom and felt that it represented state presumption of what was in the patient's best interests. In addition, many patients have become aware that GPs were incentivised by prescribing and performance targets, so that when disagreements occur over the best management of a patient's condition, suspicion arises that the GP is motivated by financial reward rather than the optimum treatment. There is evidence that the population health gains attributable to QuOF were small.[6]

A parallel movement affecting doctors' accountability in the last 20 years has been the rise of clinical governance. Historically, there was an unwritten assumption that all doctors were excellent – the mistakes in medicine were acts of god rather than due to ignorance or negligence or system failure. The demise of deference towards the medical profession has meant that patients no longer accept adverse outcomes with equanimity. Among the drivers for the introduction of systems of clinical governance were the scandals of the 1990s (such as the death rates in the paediatric surgery department at Bristol Royal Infirmary, the Rodney Ledward case, and that of Harold Shipman) and the seminal document produced by the Chief Medical Officer for Great Britain, *A First Class Service*, 1998.[7] A subsequent report by the Chief Medical Officer recognised that the NHS had a 'blame culture' and that the natural instinct of clinicians faced with things going wrong was to excuse or obfuscate.[8] Clinical governance can be defined as 'a framework through which NHS organisations are accountable for continuously improving the quality of their services and safeguarding high standards of care, by creating an environment in which excellence in clinical care will flourish'[7] and its scope and complexity is far too great for detailed discussion here. Its main implication is that doctors now have to make the measure and improvement of quality of care central to their work. As a result, they devote far greater portions of their time to activities such as clinical audit, significant event analysis, morbidity and mortality meetings and dealing with complaints. While this is only right and proper in a twenty-first-century healthcare system, there is no doubt that this also has a significant impact on the delivery of care. Workforce planning in both primary and secondary care has not, in the view of these authors, taken this into account, so that clinicians find themselves stretched more than ever before in service delivery while simultaneously being expected to maintain the quality of that service as part of their working routine. However, clinical governance is not merely an internal audit of whether and how things go wrong in healthcare (as inevitably they will from time to time): it also implies a degree of openness about processes and outcomes that clinicians were not previously used to. This was summed up by Sir Liam Donaldson, speaking at the launch of the World Alliance for Patient Safety in Washington DC on 27 October 2004 as: 'To err is human, to cover up is unforgivable, and to fail to learn is inexcusable'.[9]

It is also apparent that governments of both political shades of the last 2 decades or so have been able to use the governance agenda, and in particular the need for the collection of data on waiting times, hospital-acquired infections, post-operative morbidity and mortality and so forth, to drive an element of competition into an otherwise centralised and uniform NHS. Hospitals, primary care trusts and individual general practices are forced to participate in the publication of data about themselves covering everything from the length of time to wait for an appointment, to the death rate associated with a particular procedure. It can be argued that greater transparency is valuable for patients and that it rewards higher-quality standards with both recognition and increased *business*. However, there is evidence that NHS organisations can *game* the system in the collection of such statistics, and in many cases so-called league tables of data are not necessarily comparing like with like.[10]

Faced with this new environment of targets, league tables, satisfaction surveys and so on, what should general practices, community and hospital trusts do? In our view, the essential elements for coping are engagement and systems. Clinician leaders and managers need to find ways of ensuring that clinical and non-clinical team members are aware of the ways in which the organisation is judged and that they attach priority to achieving such measures. Financial incentives are of limited value, as most employees of the NHS come to it through motives such as altruism, interest in science or the value of human contact, but they can sometimes be useful as a way of recognising the effort involved in hitting targets. A systems-based approach is also needed – successful organisations construct processes whereby it is easier for individuals to *do the right thing,* but they also detect and remediate early when there have been lapses.

This chapter opened with an excerpt from an account of the aloof attitudes of the medical profession in the 1930s. Those entering the profession today as new doctors would do well to read it. As they embark on a career bound by clinical governance, performance review and targets, they may not realise just how far we have come.

REFERENCES

1. Cronin AJ. *The Citadel.* New York, NY: Grosset & Dunlap; 1937.
2. Cronin AJ. Interview given in *The Daily Express.* 20 July 1937.
3. Professor the Lord Darzi of Denham KBE. *High Quality Care for All.* London: Department of Health; 2008. Available at: www.dh.gov.uk/en/ Publicationsandstatistics/Publications/PublicationsPolicyAndGuidance/ DH_085825 (accessed 18 September 2012).
4. General Medical Council (GMC). *Good Medical Practice.* London: GMC; 2006. Available at: www.gmc-uk.org/guidance/good_medical_practice.asp (accessed 18 September 2012).
5. Dixon A, Khachatryan A, Wallace A, *et al. Impact of Quality and Outcomes Framework on Health Inequalities.* London: The King's Fund; 2011. Available at: www.kingsfund.org.uk/publications/impact-quality-and-outcomes-framework-health-inequalities (accessed 18 October 2012).
6. Fleetcroft R, Parekh-Bhurke S, Howe AC, *et al.* The UK pay-for-performance programme in primary care: estimation of population mortality reduction. *Br J Gen Pract.* 2010; **60**(578): 649–54.
7. Department of Health. *A First Class Service: quality in the new NHS.* London: Department of Health; 1998. Available at: www.dh.gov.uk/en/Publications andstatistics/Publications/PublicationsPolicyAndGuidance/DH_4006902 (accessed 18 September 2012).
8. Department of Health. *An Organisation with a Memory: report of an expert group on learning from adverse events in the NHS chaired by the Chief Medical Officer.* London: The Stationery Office; 2000. Available at: www.dh.gov.uk/ prod_consum_dh/groups/dh_digitalassets/@dh/@en/documents/digitalas-set/dh_4065086.pdf (accessed 18 October 2012).
9. Department of Health. *CMO Quotes: patient safety.* London: Department of Health; 2009. Available at: http://webarchive.nationalarchives.gov.uk/+/ www.dh.gov.uk/en/Aboutus/MinistersandDepartmentLeaders/Chief MedicalOfficer/CMOPublications/QuoteUnquote/DH_4102570 (accessed 18 October 2012).
10. Adab P, Rouse AM, Mohammed MA, *et al.* Performance league tables: the NHS deserves better. *BMJ.* 2002; **324**(7329): 95–8.

CHAPTER 7

The 'expert patient' and the internet

Andrea Stöckl

INTRODUCTION

This chapter deals with the question of what constitutes expertise and experience in the era of the internet in relation to the changing roles of doctors. Information-seeking behaviour has changed rapidly over the last 20 years, and this phenomenon influences not only the relationship between doctor and patients but also ideas concerning healthcare seeking and well-being in general. The internet has changed the way in which patients can gain easy access to what was previously seen as expert knowledge and only privy to a small circle of experts. The shared decision-making model, which proposes that patients make an informed decision about their medical treatment together with a medical professional, has simultaneously evolved. One could argue that this has turned patients into proto-professionals who now have to have a certain level of expertise in order to consent to medical treatment.[1] This 'professionalisation' of the patient has caused a change in how expertise and experience are defined, and it has also led to patient advocacy groups who have a big presence on the internet. Patient advocacy groups claim that the experience of suffering makes them equally equipped and gives them the right to give advice on medical matters.[2,3] Research funders and grant-giving bodies also include lay experts in their decision-making process and request that their knowledge is included in research matters. At the core of all these developments lies a new definition of what constitutes knowledge, expertise and experience. Following recent sociological debates on the changing notion of these terms, this chapter discusses the way in which these terms have underpinned current debates on the role of expert patients, patient advocates and the role that the internet plays in these developments. There are two social trends at work in this development: first, there are changes in the way in which the doctor–patient relationship is reconceptualised; second, there is a general trend in society to question scientific expertise, not just medical expertise and medical knowledge.[4] Social scientists who study the relationship between science and society,[4] have already pointed to the fact that scientific knowledge is in general less well regarded in the new millennium than it was in the postwar era, when scientific progress was unquestionably a good thing. The general feeling that we live in an age of uncertainty,[5] and that the public has lost trust in expertise, especially in medical expertise, characterise these developments. The inception of the internet as a tool for information giving and finding has certainly accelerated this phenomenon. The concepts of 'expertise' and 'experience' are key in this shift of professional power and knowledge and will now be considered in relation to patients.

WHAT IS AN EXPERT PATIENT?

Sociologists such as Collins and Evans[6] define an 'expert' as a person who possesses acquired knowledge which distinguishes their knowledge from other people in their social environment. With this knowledge and its application, expert status can be claimed within that social environment.[6] Flyvbjerg[7] refers to the five-step model of expertise development to distinguish an expert from a learner: a learner starts out as a novice in a field, then he or she moves on to being an advanced beginner, to a competent performer, a proficient performer and, eventually, some master the skills and become experts. What is crucial in this definition of expertise is the fact that becoming an expert necessarily implies following a trajectory in order to master specific skills. An expert is someone who synchronically and holistically makes decisions by being intuitively and rationally aware of their strategies and actions. Expertise is a performance, which seems effortless to the onlooker.[7] However, the term 'expert' is commonly used in a non-technical sense. Often, calling someone an expert is a political decision and not a description of their levels of skill. From a historical perspective, expert status has been attributed to the 'traditional' medical doctor, who was usually from the elite classes of society. Expert knowledge was kept within this elite class. The boundaries between experts and non-experts were clearly defined. From the perspective of political discourse the notion of the expert patient has more to do with a political decision and less with a description of the skills and knowledge of the patient. The National Health Service expert patient initiative has used this notion of expertise strategically. For example when the notion of the expert patient was first introduced in National Health Service policy in the early 2000s, the emphasis was mostly on management skills and less on knowledge and information giving. The policy stated that patients could develop the necessary self-management skills to improve their quality of life, and this in turn would also have an impact on disease management.[8] This new role of the patient can also be described as a 'proto-professional'; someone who is not a fatalistic believer in God's Will, but a person who constantly observes their health status, fully aware of the new medical technologies that allow for self-monitoring. They work closely together with a health professional in maintaining a healthy status quo. Choice, enterprise and self-actualisation are some aspects of these new health regimens.[1] This development has been put into a wider context of a future society, especially for the United States healthcare context, in which it is predicted that there will be no more doctors, and that primary healthcare will vanish by 2025.[9] The healthcare systems in the United Kingdom and continental Europe certainly differ from the United States system, but some of their predictions might ring true also for a European context.

Researchers have predicted major developments which will change the doctor–patient relationship as we know it at the moment.[9] For instance, the epidemiological transition – that is, the change in patterns of morbidity – has an impact on the doctor–patient relationship. People no longer die predominantly from infectious diseases; they live longer, yet they suffer from lifestyle-related chronic and degenerative diseases. The role of the doctor changes from being the 'hero' who saves lives to the advisor who manages chronic disorders. Status loss goes hand in hand with this development, as the doctor joins ranks with other healthcare professionals in order to manage diseases but not cure them. A further aspect that changes healthcare is the fallout from the unintended consequences of clinical guidelines. Contemporary clinical advice is lagging behind the needs of ever-increasing complex disorders. Clinical guidelines purport to give advice according to the gold standard of evidence-based medicine, but they presume that a patient has a single disorder that can be treated according to this gold standard. However, the complexity of disorders is hardly ever taken into account. Increasingly formulaic care no longer accounts for the complexity of certain disorders such as rheumatoid arthritis or type 2 diabetes. Interventions that are less complex could also be delivered by an appropriately trained health-care worker, or indeed a computer, which makes a diagnosis and prescribes and monitors medication. McKinlay and Marceau[9] predict that monitoring will increasingly happen over the internet, thus making the primary care doctor obsolete. Indeed, groups of internet users who gather on the basis of their somatic properties already exist. The measurement of these properties and the communication in specifically formed online groups is at the core of their interest. The internet has been the subject of research by an increasing number of social and political scientists since it became a mass phenomenon in the early 1990s. Their findings have confirmed that people are turning in increasing numbers to the internet in order to find information that they previously would have sought among family and friends, or to which they did not have access in the first place. For the remainder of this chapter, the reasons people use the internet for their healthcare-seeking behaviour will be discussed.

HEALTH, ILLNESS AND DISEASE ON THE INTERNET

Online behaviour usually follows a trajectory. The initial step is simple information-seeking behaviour: someone feels that something is wrong with them; they have been given a diagnosis by a healthcare professional; they do not understand this information, so they type the symptom or the diagnosis into a search engine to gain a better understanding of their condition. Some people do not stop there but rather move on to following and/or becoming part of an online community, or they use the internet for monitoring their illness, their health and their well-being.[10] Once they have established themselves in a community, they start communicating: narrating their experiences, writing a blog about their predicaments and their coping strategies, or using the wider public as a tool to monitor their progress in lifestyle decisions such as losing weight. Each of these behaviours will be discussed in the following sections.

Information-seeking behaviour

Information-seeking behaviour on the internet is one of the most common activities. It is estimated that more people go online in order to seek health advice than visit a health professional or a general practitioner.[10-12] The foremost reasons for people to go online is that they feel embarrassed about their symptoms and fear that they will be stigmatised.[12] The symptoms might be in the body, such as urinary incontinency or herpes warts; however, most people go online to look up conditions such as anxiety or depression.[12] Furthermore, research on adolescents showed they go online more often than older people.[13] A study comparing students' healthcare-seeking in the United States and the United Kingdom confirmed that the internet was their primary source for information regarding their healthcare. The students also found the information salient, yet they were aware of the trustworthiness issues of the information. This contrasts with research on parents of children who had been diagnosed with paediatric cancer in the United States[14]; parents preferred to trust the actual advice they were given by their consultants rather than the information they found on the internet. Their reasons for not trusting the information on the internet in an acute crisis was that they feared what they might find online, or they were uncertain about the accuracy of the information. They also felt that they were overloaded with specific information that they could not make sense of. The experience of not being able to make sense, to give a meaning to experience, is what usually leads people to the second step in their online behaviour: joining communities of sufferers to share experiences.

Virtual communities

A second aspect of online health and illness advice seeking is joining a community. Online communities of people who share their predicaments are mostly populated by people who first logged on to the internet in order to seek information but found that there is a whole world of new communities out there waiting for them. Some of these communities are dedicated to sharing the experience of suffering; some develop into political agents in their own right. Dumit[15] has described online forums for sufferers from rare disorders as spaces in which people campaign for 'illnesses you have to fight to get', such as chronic fatigue syndrome, or multiple chemical sensitivities. Endometriosis[16] or Morgellon's disease[17] are more examples of these contested illnesses. Online communities can also turn into spaces for political debates: for instance, communities that defend the right to be 'neuro-diverse' instead of being labelled as 'autistic'.[3] Some of these online communities have grown into citizenship rights movements, such as some disability rights movements, and here especially the autism rights movements in some European countries. Research on autism organisations in France shows how parents concerned with the stigmatising diagnosis of their autistic children tried to change the treatment of their children against the dominating ideas of the psychiatrists who were in charge of developing protocols for treatment.[3] The parents' association tried to change the treatment to the United States model, which was more about collaboration between medical professionals, parents and their autistic children. Parents wanted to be seen as partners of their children, they wanted to be trained in behavioural methodology in order to be in a better position to deal with them, but the powerful psychiatric domination in France prevented them from achieving these goals. Psychiatrists still treat autistic children from a psychodynamic perspective, rather than seeing autism as a genetic disease of diversity. The internet allowed the parents to organise themselves and turn their plight into a political movement, one of the last citizenship rights movement is the disability movement, as the researcher argues. The internet has helped to redefine the identity of the people belonging to these online communities. Members of these groups want to be seen as people with a different cognitive mode of functioning, not as 'people with autism'. Only the future can tell in which direction the political discourse about autism, disability and citizenship rights will lead.

Another aspect of community building on the internet is that of social support and social capital, for situations in which the extended family and friends would have given real life support but are no longer there to do this. Motherhood, for instance, is such an exceptional situation in which women find themselves these days without the support of their own mothers or friends who could provide them with much needed advice. Online groups dedicated to parents' support can provide their participants with emotional and instrumental support and with community building and protection.[18]

In the previous paragraphs, the usage of the internet by people who have been diagnosed with a rare disease or those with a contested disease, or those who have children with rare genetic disorders has been discussed. Information seeking and community building of these groups all follow similar behaviour patterns. One example for a citizenship rights movement is the HIV/AIDS media activism groups[19] who used the internet to campaign for a better understanding of their autobiographies and their expertise that resulted from being diagnosed with a disease that is severely stigmatised. The internet was used in order to make the private trouble of people with HIV/AIDS open to the public sphere. It served as a midway between a self-promoted newsletter and the television. Researchers who examined the rise and the diversification of websites that deal with HIV/AIDS infection noted that the second wave of these websites were more about HIV infection and not so much about having to live and cope with AIDS. There was thus a significant shift towards sharing expertise in how to live with HIV and how not to develop full-blown AIDS. Autobiographical accounts were mixed with giving expert advice on living with HIV. The expertise was about the history of the epidemic, what to expect after being diagnosed, what to expect from drug treatment, links to other websites and how to deal with health professionals. Many of the people living with HIV/AIDS who created these websites prided themselves in their knowledge and their expertise. They also pointed out that their expertise was not professional but that it came from having experienced the aftermath of having been diagnosed with this stigmatised disease.[19] Expertise in this sense is used as sharing lived experience, educating other people who are or are not diagnosed with the disease, and educating the general public. Lay knowledge is promoted to communicate more effectively with health professionals.

In this section on online illness communities one more aspect of this phenomenon will be discussed: parents who seek advice about their children's genetic conditions. Information seeking about the often difficult to understand technical and medical terminology of genetics brings these parents to seek for information online, and they subsequently form online communities. The difference to the communities discussed earlier – that is, the citizenship rights movements of parents with autistic children or of people living with AIDS – is that these parents find it easier to cope with their everyday lives outside of the internet realm. Research on parents who use the internet to find out more about their children's rare diseases[20] shows that they manage to adjust better to extremely stressful situations after having consulted and shared experiences with other parents online. Becoming knowledgeable about a disease and sharing difficulties of adjusting is thus essential for a better life with rare genetic disorders offline.[20]

Embodied virtual spaces

When the internet first became a mass phenomenon, there was a lot of theoretical debate on whether real and virtual space was divided. Was the online representation only a 'psychological' disembodied sphere? Ever since then, it has become obvious that the mind–body divide does not hold up to scrutiny and that the virtual space is as much embodied as 'real' life is. Writing about bodily disorders or bodily harm – or, indeed, enjoying a completely invented embodied self – has become an everyday occurrence. The third aspect of how people use the internet for negotiating health and illness is thus the so-called 'blogosphere', which denominates a virtual space in which an individual writes about experiencing their bodies as if it was a diary, although the diary is open to the public. Many of these open diaries deal with 'embodied' pain, such as injuring the body in self-harm[21] or the challenges of being stigmatised for suffering from anorexia.[22] Other aspects of dealing with painful embodiment are blogs on which people negotiate their suicidal thoughts and their desire to eliminate the body and the self completely.[23] On a slightly healthier note, there has been a rapid growth in blogging activities related to the notoriously difficult activity of losing weight.[24] Many bloggers use their blogs to 'keep them going' (i.e. to be accountable to their achievements and not to lose track of their goals). The bloggers construct a different self as their bodies transform, but they also face the difficulties of negotiating privacy and disclosure issues. Painful embodiment, which means having a body with which the person is not happy, seems to be difficult to negotiate in everyday 'real life' in which a lot of people feel stigmatised and ostracised; yet the blogosphere and online communities offer a semi-public space in which the self and the body can be discussed and sometimes reunited in a novel way, thus allowing for a better adjustment in non-virtual spaces.

CONCLUSION

The development of online healthcare (and illness-) seeking behaviour has of course not gone unnoticed by health professionals, and their response has been varied. Researchers on the consequence of internet health research have classified these reactions as celebratory, concerned and contingent.[10] It has been argued that most social scientists and policy analysts welcomed the lay usage of the internet for health purposes as an opportunity of empowerment and fostering patient and lay expertise. However, a second perspective, mostly coming from the medical professionals, is that of the concerned professional, which ranges from being concerned to describing internet healthcare-seeking behaviour as 'dangerous'. These views are mostly expressed about incorrect healthcare advice and the additional demand it will generate for healthcare professionals, such as general practitioners, who will have to cope with patients who consider themselves well informed and who cite every study they found on the internet. However, a third way of making decisions about the information found on the internet has also been described. Most patients, it is argued, can make 'a reasonable assessment'[10] of the information they find on the internet. Laypeople are perfectly capable of distinguishing what is good for them and what is not. This view comes from the argument that the novelty of the internet has worn off already. In the 1990s, people used the internet in a much more trusting way than they do in the new millennium; the usage of the internet has become embedded in everyday life.

Sociologists have routinely described this era as the information age; but with the idea of information also comes the idea of reflexivity.[25] Reflexive modernisation stands for the trend which seems to follow otherwise disparate aspects of modern life in that it describes the uncertainty, unpredictability and instability of contemporary economic and private life. People's lives have become much less predictable than they used to be. The person who is exposed to these circumstances develops a reflexive self. This means that constant control and self-monitoring of actions and thoughts has become mandatory.[25] A lot of reflective resources have sprung up in order to make the permanent self-control and reflexivity easier: therapy, self-help manuals, TV and magazine articles. The internet is just one of these new technologies that allows the twenty-first-century citizen to self-monitor every aspect of their lives, including health and well-being. However, uncertainty and unpredictability, which is by now an agreed aspect of any scientific endeavour, also affects the lay expertise. The changing notion of expertise and the way in which patients are turned into proto-professionals who have to, willingly or not, participate in the decision-making of their healthcare was discussed previously. This development is probably here to stay. Future primary healthcare will thus have to take the expert patient into account as much as the expert patient will have to take into account that doctors expect them to be well informed.

REFERENCES

1. Novas C, Rose N. Genetic risk and the birth of the somatic individual. *Eco Soc.* 2000; 29(4): 485–513.
2. Barker KK, Galardi TR. Dead by 50: lay expertise and breast cancer screening. *Soc Sci Med.* 2011; 72(8): 1351–8.
3. Chamak B. Autism and social movements: French parents' associations and

international autistic individuals' organisations. *Sociol Health Illn*. 2008; **30**(1): 76–96.

4. Nowotny H, Scott P, Gibbons M. *Re-Thinking Science: knowledge and the public in an age of uncertainty*. Cambridge: Polity Press; 2001.

5. O'Neill O. *Autonomy and Trust in Bioethics*. Cambridge: Cambridge University Press; 2002.

6. Collins H, Evans R. *Rethinking Expertise*. Chicago, IL: University of Chicago Press; 2007.

7. Flyvbjerg B. *Making Social Science Matter*. Cambridge: Cambridge University Press; 2001.

8. www.nhs.uk/NHSEngland/AboutNHSservices/doctors/Pages/expert-patients-programme.aspx (accessed 4 February 2013).

9. McKinlay J, Marceau L. When there is no doctor: reasons for the disappearance of primary care physicians in the US during the early 21st century. *Soc Sci Med*. 2008; **67**(10): 1481–91.

10. Nettleton S, Burrows R, O'Malley L. The mundane realities of the everyday lay use of the internet for health, and their consequences for media convergence. *Sociol Health Illn*. 2005; **27**(7): 972–92.

11. Cotten SR, Gupta SS. Characteristics of online and offline health information seekers and factors that discriminate between them. *Soc Sci Med*. 2004; **59**(9): 1795–806.

12. Berger M, Wagner TH, Baker LC. Internet use and stigmatized illness. *Soc Sci Med*. 2005; **61**(8): 1821–7.

13. Gray NJ, Klein JD, Noyce PR, *et al*. Health information-seeking behaviour in adolescence: the place of the internet. *Soc Sci Med*. 2005; **60**(7): 1467–78.

14. Gage EA, Panagakis C. The devil you know: parents seeking information online for paediatric cancer. *Sociol Health Illn*. 2012; **34**(3): 444–58.

15. Dumit J. Illnesses you have to fight to get: facts as forces in uncertain, emergent illnesses. *Soc Sci Med*. 2006; **62**(3): 577–90.

16. Whelan E. 'No one agrees except for those of us who have it': endometriosis patients as an epistemological community. *Sociol Health Illn*. 2007; **29**(7): 957–82.

17. Fair B. Morgellons: contested illness, diagnostic compromise and medicalisation. *Sociol Health Illn*. 2010; **32**(4): 597–612.

18. Drentea P, Moren-Cross JL. Social capital and social support on the web: the case of an internet mother site. *Sociol Health Illn*. 2005; **27**(7): 920–43.

19. Gillett J. Media activism and internet use by people with HIV/AIDS. *Sociol Health Illn*. 2003; **25**(6): 608–24.

20. Gundersen T. 'One wants to know what a chromosome is': the internet as a coping resource when adjusting to life parenting a child with a rare genetic disorder. *Soc Health Illn*. 2011; **33**(1): 81–95.

21. Klineberg E. The tender cut: inside the hidden world of self-injury. *Sociol Health Illn*. 2012; **34**(5): 806–7.

22. Rich E. Anorexic dis(connection): managing anorexia as an illness and an identity. *Sociol Health Illn*. 2006; **28**(3): 284–305.

23. Horne J, Wiggins S. Doing being 'on the edge': managing the dilemma of being authentically suicidal in an online forum. *Sociol Health Illn.* 2009; 31(2): 170–84.

24. Leggatt-Cook C, Chamberlain K. Blogging for weight loss: personal account-ability, writing selves, and the weight-loss blogosphere. *Sociol Health Illn.* 2011; 34(7): 963–77.

25. Giddens A. *Modernity and Self-Identity: self and society in the late modern age.* Cambridge: Polity Press; 1991.

CHAPTER 8

Regulation and revalidation

Richard Young and Krishna Sethia

INTRODUCTION

All professions rely on a bond of trust between their members and the public. For doctors, this trust means that the public must have confidence that individual practitioners offer them the highest clinical standards of care and that these practitioners behave with integrity. Unfortunately, a series of high-profile scandals in the past 25 years has eroded that trust and it has therefore become incumbent on the profession to attempt to restore confidence. Little more than a decade or so ago, there was a presumption that once licensed to practise by the General Medical Council (GMC) a doctor would remain on the register indefinitely unless removed or suspended as the result of an investigation into fitness to practise or professional misconduct. By the end of the 1990s this was no longer acceptable. The announcement of revalidation in 1999[1,2] signalled the single biggest change in the regulation of doctors in the United Kingdom for a generation. Thirteen years later we have reached the stage where the process can start to be implemented, with the expectation that all practising doctors will have undergone revalidation by 2016. In this chapter we examine the events and drivers that have brought this about, and we discuss why it has taken so long to be implemented.

HISTORY

The historical perspective is that medicine in the United Kingdom has been, and ostensibly remains, a self-regulating profession. The 'General Council of Medical Education and Registration of the United Kingdom', as it was first known, came into being as a result of the

Medical Act 1858[3] and with the primary purpose of establishing a register of qualified medical practitioners. Those not on the register were excluded from working in specific areas such as hospitals, the military services, and societies for affording mutual relief in sickness. An interesting consequence of the Act was that it required the recognition of foreign medical degrees for admission to the register and thereby led to the registration of the United Kingdom's first female doctor, Elizabeth Blackwell, who, having been unable to enter a medical school in the United Kingdom, had qualified in the United States. The original Council was made up entirely of representatives of medical and surgical colleges, other professional bodies such as the Society of Apothecaries, and the senior universities of the time, and so by definition was drawn from the profession itself. Although it had the power to erase the names of doctors from the register in cases of conviction of 'felony and misdemeanor' and being guilty of 'infamous conduct',[3] there were no sanctions for cases of lesser offence. Indeed, there was no mention in the Act as such of any role other than the admission of doctors to the right to practise in the United Kingdom. Even in 1858 it was recognised that the practice of medicine was a matter of judgement and opinion, and it was expressly stated that erasure from the register could not be solely on the grounds of the practitioner 'having adopted any theory of medicine or surgery'.[3]

The first formal recognition of a disciplinary role for the General Medical Council came in the Medical Act 1950, which also conferred upon it officially the name by which the Council had been known for some time. The principle of regulation of the profession by the profession remained largely intact; the membership of the council was to be widened to 47 members, 11 of these directly elected from the profession, and lay members were included for the first time. However, it was clear from the *British Medical Journal*'s report of the new Act[4] that the expectation was that these posts would be filled by Members of Parliament, so the GMC could hardly be said to have become representative of the wider population. Disciplinary cases could be heard by a quorum of as little as five of the 18-strong disciplinary committee; however, for the first time a right of appeal against the decisions of the GMC was enshrined in law.

The later history of the GMC's role in ensuring good standards in medical practice and dealing with practitioners who did not meet those standards is not a happy one. The decades between 1970 and 1999 saw increasing public and professional[5] criticism of the GMC's composition and effectiveness in dealing with poorly performing doctors. This was compounded by a succession of high-profile cases in the 1990s and early 2000s,[6] which left the public and media[7] with a strong feeling that the regulatory framework was not fit for purpose. The culmination of this was the Department of Health report *Good Doctors, Safer Patients* in 2006 by the then Chief Medical Officer, Sir Liam Donaldson,[8] who characterised the state of affairs thus: 'the General Medical Council seems to be neither highly valued nor fully trusted by either the general public or the medical profession'. His report drew heavily on the conclusions of the inquiries into the practice of Dr Harold Shipman, a city general practitioner, who was convicted of multiple murder in 2000. Most of his victims were elderly women, killed by injections of diamorphine. These inquiries, led by Dame Janet Smith, were highly critical of the GMC. In particular, the inquiries identified that revalidation, as then proposed by the GMC, would be unlikely to have prevented Shipman's activities. According to Donaldson, revalidation needed to go further than demonstrating simple engagement with the process of annual appraisal: 'it should be patient centred, promote improvement of standards, root out bad or sub-standard practice and be rigorous.' Meanwhile, the government pressed on with the adoption of a civil rather than criminal standard of proof in cases of misconduct or poor performance. Although this was seen to redress the balance of power in favour of patients, it was criticised as unfair to doctors, whose livelihoods and professional reputations were at stake.[9]

REVALIDATION

Initial suggestions were that revalidation should occur in two parts: relicensing and revalidation, being the responsibilities of the GMC and the Royal Colleges, respectively. This division was soon abandoned for one process under GMC control, but for many years the various Royal Colleges have been working on a succession of specialist interpretations of the requirements for revalidation, to the increasing bewilderment of their members. During this period, somewhat controversially, the concept that revalidation should include a test of knowledge was abandoned and it became clear that the process would depend solely upon successful completion of annual enhanced appraisals. It remains to be seen whether this lack of a formal exam, which is common in other countries (e.g. US boards), will reduce public confidence in the process.

It was perhaps inevitable that the implementation of such a

major regulatory change affecting over 130 000 doctors would be a prolonged affair. The combination of intense debate in the medical media, a change of government in 2010 to a political party who were committed to a major structural reform of the National Health Service, and the slow pace of centralised bureaucracy has meant that it is only in 2013 that the first 20% of doctors will become revalidated. Revalidation for the remaining 80% will be completed by 2016.

To achieve revalidation, a network of 'responsible officers' (ROs) has been created. Every doctor is obliged to identify his or her RO, who would normally be a senior member (e.g. medical director, postgraduate dean) of the employing organisation for which the individual spends the majority of his or her working time. The RO has a responsibility to maintain records on all doctors within his or her jurisdiction and to ensure that the organisation has a robust governance mechanism that will detect poor performance. Where deficiencies in practice are identified, organisations must provide remedial training whenever possible. Following completion of a series (normally 5 years) of annual appraisals, the RO should thus be in a position to make an informed recommendation for revalidation to the GMC.

The evidence upon which enhanced appraisal can be satisfactorily completed is now summarised by the GMC in *Supporting Information for Appraisal and Revalidation*.[10] This document covers all specialties and stipulates that all doctors will be required to submit six types of evidence in order to be revalidated. The role of the specialist colleges will be to advise doctors on what sort of evidence is relevant and appropriate to their discipline, and to provide structures and frameworks to help support the collection of that evidence – for example, the Royal College of General Practitioners Revalidation e-Portfolio.

The six types of evidence required are:
1. Continuing professional development
2. Quality improvement activity
3. Significant events
4. Feedback from colleagues
5. Feedback from patients (where applicable)
6. Review of complaints and compliments.

CONTINUING PROFESSIONAL DEVELOPMENT

It has been generally accepted for some time that no medical practitioner can rely purely on the knowledge and skills obtained in their years of postgraduate training; new treatments, better evidence and altered demands of the role mean that all doctors need to update themselves. Continuing professional development (CPD) implies an active process of reflection on learning needs, strategic planning of how such needs will be met, and demonstrating how new knowledge and skills are incorporated into practice. The latest GMC guidance indicates that practitioners will need to demonstrate that these elements are present in at least a proportion of the educational activity in which they engage. It will not suffice, for example, for a doctor to simply state that they have spent 50 hours reading the *British Medical Journal* in the past year. This may present more of a challenge to doctors who qualified, say, more than 10 years ago – many of this generation were not taught principles of reflective practice and may have a somewhat haphazard approach to acquisition of new understandings. Portfolios, reflective diaries, practitioner groups and journal clubs can all help, but, again, these are all activities that may not come naturally to isolated senior clinicians. Additionally, the increasing pressures of service delivery mean that CPD can be squeezed out. Medical managers need to allocate time to activities that support CPD and recognise that they can improve quality of care, keep clinicians motivated and help them retain their licence to practise. The Royal Colleges representing the various specialties also have a role in ensuring that doctors collect relevant and appropriate CPD evidence. The Royal College of General Practitioners, in particular, has developed an electronic portfolio to aid the collection of CPD evidence and is heavily promoting its own 'Essential Knowledge Updates' as a way of accumulating the necessary credits.

QUALITY IMPROVEMENT ACTIVITY

Health organisations worldwide have realised that quality improvement is an essential goal, not only to improve outcomes for individual patients but also to ensure the financial viability of their service. For revalidation every doctor needs to be able to demonstrate that he or she is involved in improving the quality of care. At its simplest this might involve contributing outcome data to local or national audits and using the results of these audits to implement change in practice. Further examples of quality improvement may involve the organised use of scientific quantitative or qualitative data to advance care. In the United Kingdom the government has set a series of quality priorities and has started to use the commissioning process to ensure adherence to national standards – that is, healthcare providers will only be paid for services that offer the required standard of care.

SIGNIFICANT EVENTS

Significant events are defined as 'any unintended or unexpected event, which could or did lead to harm of one or more patients'.[10] Through the work of the National Patient Safety Agency, established in 2001, it has become routine practice in many hospital departments and general practices to discuss 'near misses', 'adverse events', 'serious incidents' and 'never events' as these are variously known. The intention is to identify ways in which systems can be improved, to reduce risk, and learning can take place to ensure that clinicians are aware of risks. However, significant event meetings run the risk of being viewed by management as a form of performance management, or of being confused with disciplinary procedures. It is not surprising, therefore, that some clinicians view this area with suspicion and that getting candid engagement, rather than defensiveness, can be difficult. However, if clinicians know that what they discuss in significant event meetings will be kept within their team, used for educational purposes and not as a means of punishment and control, they are more likely to engage. Doctors undergoing revalidation will need to demonstrate such engagement, and they will not need to fear that they are required to publicly own up to adverse outcomes.

FEEDBACK FROM COLLEAGUES AND PATIENTS

Feedback from colleagues and patients may represent the largest cultural shift of all for a profession that has historically been somewhat above criticism. The tendency for doctors to be put on pedestals by laypeople, allied health professions and junior colleagues led to presumptions of infallibility. During the period of the most intense criticism of the GMC, medicine in the United Kingdom ran a very real risk of losing its self-regulatory status; the profession has had to embrace greater transparency and the notion that doctors should accept and respond to feedback on their performance. The concept of 360-degree feedback (i.e. ratings of performance provided from the full range of perspectives surrounding the individual) has been familiar to managers in the commercial sector since the 1990s, but it has only gained acceptance in healthcare more recently. However, since the inception of the Foundation Programme (the initial 2 years of postgraduate training for newly qualified doctors) in 2005[11] and the workplace-based assessment for Membership of the Royal College of General Practitioners in 2006, it has been routine practice for general practitioner trainees to submit evidence from patient and colleague surveys, and it seems likely that other Royal Colleges will follow suit.

Seeing their junior colleagues undergoing 360-degree feedback may well have familiarised longer-serving doctors with the idea that they might be subject to the same process.

REVIEW OF COMPLAINTS AND COMPLIMENTS

Review of complaints and compliments is another potentially contentious area. Given the huge number of consultations, procedures and decisions taking place daily in the National Health Service, what is surprising is how few complaints there are. Complaints, particularly those about an individual doctor, can be devastating personally, and many doctors would rather deal with them as quickly as possible and move on. The prospect of having to rake over negative feedback and demonstrate evidence of reflection on it is not an enticing one. Thankfully for many doctors, it is likely that in a 5-year cycle there will be little negative and some positive to discuss. However, the random occurrence of complaints and their tendency to cluster may find some doctors having to consider a 5-year period with a lot on the negative side of the balance sheet.

CONCLUSIONS

In summary, it would appear that the GMC is moving to attempt to demonstrate that doctors keep themselves up to date, reflect upon mistakes and near misses to improve patient care, and remain fit to practise. It is to be hoped that the habits required of CPD, regular reflection on practice and being transparent about needs for improvement will encourage weaker doctors to aspire to the standards of the best. Only time will tell whether this hope is realistic. It is clear that revalidation will occupy considerable amounts of doctors' time, and, in order for them to remain engaged with the process, employing organisations will need to maintain fair and robust mechanisms for evaluating performance and dealing with concerns. At the same time, the GMC needs to demonstrate that it deals fairly with both doctors and patients.

REFERENCES

1. Southgate L, Pringle M. Revalidation in the United Kingdom: general principles based on experience in general practice. *BMJ.* 1999; 319(7218): 1180–3.
2. Department of Health. *Supporting Doctors, Protecting Patients: a consultation paper.* London: Department of Health; 1999. Available at: www.dh.gov.uk/en/Publicationsandstatistics/Publications/PublicationsPolicyAndGuidance/DH_4005688 (accessed 12 August 2012).

3. Medical Act 1858. Available at: www.legislation.gov.uk/ukpga/Vict/21-22/90/contents (accessed 11 September 2012).

4. The Medical Act. *Br Med J*. 1950; **2**(4674): 337–8.

5. GMS Committee. From the GMS Committee: composition of the General Medical Council. *Br Med J (Clin Res Ed)*. 1983; **286**(6376): 1526–8.

6. Dixon-Woods M, Yeung K, Bosk CL. Why is U.K. medicine no longer a self-regulating profession? The role of scandals involving 'bad apple' doctors. *Soc Sci Med*. 2011; **73**(10): e1452–9.

7. Batty D. The GMC in crisis. *Society Guardian*. 2001; 29 May.

8. Donaldson L. *Good Doctors, Safer Patients*. London: Department of Health; 2006. Available at: www.dh.gov.uk/en/Publicationsandstatistics/Publications/PublicationsPolicyAndGuidance/DH_4137232 (accessed 11 September 2012).

9. Kemp S. The impact of the civil standard of proof in fitness to practise hearings. *Health Serv J*. 2008; 15 January.

10. General Medical Council (GMC). *Supporting Information for Appraisal and Revalidation*. London: GMC; 2012. Available at: www.gmc-uk.org/doctors/revalidation/revalidation_information.asp (accessed 11 September 2012).

11. Hays R. Foundation programme for newly qualified doctors. *BMJ*. 2005; **331**(7515): 465–6.

CHAPTER 9

Interprofessional practice and rank dynamics: evolving effective team collaboration through emotional, social, occupational and spiritual intelligences

Mick Collins and Susanne Lindqvist

INTRODUCTION

The last decade has witnessed a shift within health professional education, towards an increased emphasis on the importance of interprofessional practice (IPP). Key areas of development in the United Kingdom have included statements from the Department of Health (DoH)[1-4] and by professional bodies highlighting the need for effective collaboration between healthcare professionals (e.g. the General Medical Council; the Nursing and Midwifery Council).[5,6] The introduction of interprofessional learning (IPL) as part of the curricula in the majority of UK higher education institutions reflects the recognition that IPL needs to be introduced at the outset of students' education and offered throughout their careers. There is an increasing body of research evidence that IPL and IPP can be promoted effectively within the process of education and life-long learning.[7]

Educating and resourcing professionals to be adequately equipped to engage effectively within an interprofessional team is an essential component of a service ethic that ensures the best standards of delivery of care are met. However, the reality of high-pressure working environments, familiar to most healthcare professionals, produces complexities and demands that require interprofessional team members to develop new levels of operational awareness. One example concerns the understanding of, and ability to deal with, rank dynamics, which can have a powerful effect on healthcare professionals and team performance. Psychologist Arnold Mindell[8] has noted how rank can be connected to sociocultural factors such as status, or how it can be cultivated through the development of personal qualities, such as resilience or self-esteem. Rank is most frequently associated with hierarchies and power, as commonly found in top-down management structures. However, rank can also be connected to people's lived experience, like when a person exudes an aura of confidence after triumphing over adverse circumstances. Mindell has identified that we communicate our rank, overtly or covertly, through our behaviours.

The integration of rank awareness within IPL and IPP could foster new dimensions of collaborative practice within teams that is supported by its members showing abilities of emotional, social, and spiritual and occupational intelligences. The key message of this chapter is that, as members of different professions, we need to rely upon one another, and the awareness of rank dynamics can help nurture more effective working relationships.

INTERPROFESSIONAL PRACTICE: THE STATE OF THE ART AND BEYOND

There has been an increasing amount of evidence supporting the benefits of IPL and IPP in the literature over the past few decades.[9,10] Outcomes of IPL include participants doing the following:

➤ engaging an increasing knowledge base about IPL and IPP
➤ modifying professional attitudes to become more positive
➤ acquiring new knowledge and skills that facilitate effective collaboration
➤ changing behaviours if necessary
➤ optimising service delivery for the well-being of patients.

The literature still lacks robust studies that consider the wider social factors that affect interprofessional relations, as discussed in a recent editorial[11] that emphasises the *social imagination*[12] and the importance of individuals understanding how their actions affect their interactions. Within the practice setting, interactions between professionals are influenced by a number of factors, some of which are fuelled by each professional protecting his or her position. One of these factors may be the underlying rank dynamics within the work setting. In times where the National Health Service (NHS) is subjected to radical change, new thinking about ways of optimising the working environment is needed. Increasing the awareness of rank may aid this new thinking and support the fostering of team dynamics that leads to improved satisfaction, not only for patients but also for staff members within interprofessional teams.

THE IMPORTANCE OF DEVELOPING AN AWARENESS OF RANK DYNAMICS WITHIN TEAMS

The DoH publication *Breaking Through*[13] has identified the need for characteristics, attitudes and behaviours that leaders should aspire to. Some of these are referred to in the *NHS Leadership Qualities Framework: Good Practice Guide*,[14] including personal integrity, self-belief, self-awareness, self-management and a drive for improvement. Since the inception of the NHS Modernisation Agency Leadership Centre, there has been a clear mandate for the workforce to embody initiatives such as Leading an Empowered Organisation.[14] Such initiatives reflect serious attempts to create a well-led, empowered, accountable and emotionally intelligent workforce. One potential stumbling block that could impede these well-intended DoH aspirations is the overemphasis on a *drive-for-results* culture,[15] which could encourage competition rather than collaboration. It is instructive to note that research has identified how competitive interactions within organisational systems are likely to lead to the formation of dominance hierarchies[7,16] that can result in power dynamics. This is a sobering reminder of the importance of addressing power imbalances and re-affirming a more positive use of rank in order to obtain effective working relationships between professionals who truly collaborate.

To avoid the worst effects of a dominance culture in organisational systems (e.g. the dominant and the dominated[17]), it is necessary to understand the complexity of rank dynamics. Physician Pierre Morin[18] refers to rank as the way power and privileges are recognised and distributed within communities. Rank dynamics are complex[18] and the full impact of status and rank in human societies has to a great extent been ignored.[19] Arnold Mindell[20] noted that understanding rank dynamics can lead to a greater appreciation of *difference* and *diversity*, in terms of people's lived experiences. For example, a psychiatrist who works with people's mental health needs has significant educational, professional and social rank arising from their knowledge about mental health, yet a mental health service user reflects subtler understandings of rank issues, which have developed through their personal experience, their *lived experiences of recovery*. As is often the case, the service user is not credited with having managed such complex physiological, psychological, emotional and social challenges, which is a clear example of hidden rank.[21] There is a need for awareness training to help interprofessional teams understand the importance of rank.

The point is that rank, beyond status and hierarchy, can be reflected in *every* human being's life experiences. Rank can be of great value in a working culture underpinned by an appreciation and understanding of diverse perspectives. In essence, awareness of rank has the potential to contribute towards working relationships that are productive[22] and collaborative. In the context of interprofessional team working, the ability of the team to evolve principles that are coherent and meaningful to all team members is dependent upon a commitment to establish clear values that support effective working practices.[23] Here, rank awareness coheres with the use of social and emotional, as well as spiritual and occupational, intelligences in order to help unlock what we have referred to as a team's *interprofessional potential*.

ACHIEVING INTERPROFESSIONAL POTENTIAL: THE RELEVANCE OF SOCIAL AND EMOTIONAL INTELLIGENCES

Because of the importance of cultivating effective team interactions, leaders must have a clear understanding of the potential negative effects of hierarchical structures, status and power upon team functioning. Leaders are in a position to be able to inspire the sophisticated use of social and emotional intelligences in order to generate good working environments instead of investing in rigid hierarchies that create power imbalances. Bourton[24] has alluded to the possibilities of a management culture exempt from power, and has suggested that cooperation may facilitate a shift from domination by management, towards greater self-management, where all members contribute to the effective running of a team. This means that team leaders need to develop skills in self-awareness and the ability to evolve collaborative working practices that encourage the growth of appropriate collective values.[25] They must take the opportunity to develop a culture of support,[26] which includes the development of trust and confidence that everyone will work together[27] and actively participate.[28] Here, the emotional energy exchange between people can significantly affect perceptions of empowerment,[29] especially in relation to positive emotions expressed within effective teams, which are considered to be linked to increases in job satisfaction.[30] Indeed, valuing emotions within an organisation, or team, can lead to improved working practices.[31]

VIGNETTE: APPLYING SOCIAL AND EMOTIONAL INTELLIGENCES IN COLLABORATIVE PRACTICE

A healthcare assistant has worked in the same department for 20 years. The assistant is well known for voicing negative opinions about any new initiatives, making statements such as: 'we tried to implement something like this once before and it was a complete waste of time'. The assistant is a strong character who is able to influence other staff, both qualified and unqualified. The team leader observed the negative effect that this healthcare assistant was having on team morale and decided to tackle the issue. The team leader noticed that the assistant is an excellent communicator who works incredibly well with patients who are vulnerable and who need time to build up their confidence prior to being discharged from hospital. During the assistant's annual appraisal the team leader spoke about the valuable therapeutic qualities that the assistant possessed, and suggested that the work they had been doing was of great importance. Indeed, the team leader expressed the view that the assistant's name had been mentioned many times in patient satisfaction feedback. The team leader then asked the assistant if they would be happy taking more of an official role in helping the more vulnerable patients in their recovery as part of a new service improvement initiative. The assistant said that they had never had a conversation like this before and stated that it was very rewarding to be recognised for their work: 'In all of the time that I have worked here I have never really felt part of the team, managers and professionals can easily overlook the good work that people like me do'. The team leader recognised, through social and emotional intelligences, the value of the healthcare assistant's feelings of disempowerment but also the assistant's willingness to take responsibility. The leader focused on the team member's underutilised skills to strengthen the work that the team is doing.

The task of bringing rank dynamics to the forefront of team enculturation is dependent upon members valuing one another for the diverse perspectives they bring to the team. In a traditional dominance-based hierarchy, power and status imbalances can engender hostile working environments.[32] In contrast, it can be argued that the success of collaborative practices is dependent upon emotional and social intelligences. Developing and mastering such intelligences can increase the possibilities of collective problem-solving, as this type of collaboration will be based on sharing knowledge and skills from a greater pool of human resources. This could include productive exchanges of information, innovation and creativity.[32]

The role of leaders in enabling effective team functioning is paramount in modern working practices, especially where there are diverse professional viewpoints, as is the case in the modern health arena. The integration of rank awareness, based on valuing difference and diversity, can be underpinned by cultivating and using social intelligence in teams, as formulated by Daniel Goleman.[33] He argues that the key premise of social intelligence is how team members' actions and interactions have an impact on the *emotional economy* of the workforce. Goleman's[34] research into emotional intelligence, which recognises how communication and feedback is at the heart of the organisation, is based upon qualities, such as self- and social awareness to help manage relationships[35] and is closely linked to social intelligence.

The emotional environment that people work in is dependent upon valuing diversity and effective networking,[33] which can capitalise on the complex interactions between people's roles and relationships within an organisational culture.[36] However, the development of rank awareness, linked to social and emotional intelligence, requires leaders to work with teams to engage and actualise the full interprofessional potential available.

ACHIEVING INTERPROFESSIONAL POTENTIAL: THE RELEVANCE OF SPIRITUAL AND OCCUPATIONAL INTELLIGENCES

Being emotionally and socially engaged within interprofessional teams, in an intelligent manner, requires the recognition and appreciation of rank awareness to support the emergence of an effective working culture. The way that people orient themselves to the challenges of tackling complexities at work, as well as engaging and sometimes actualising their interprofessional potential, is based upon understanding the meaning and purpose that each individual invests in their working lives, and the contribution they make to the communities to which they belong. Weiss *et al.*[37] have reported that when human beings reflect on their career choice or work success, they may ask themselves what their work means to them, or whether their work serves a deeper purpose. Finding meaningful responses to such essential questions can become a spiritual task.[37] Addressing these kinds of questions within interprofessional teams may enable members to help others as well as cultivating a deeper, more sacred, view of their actions in the world.[38] The ability to use spiritual qualities in the working environment is dependent upon understanding how the parameters of human potential go beyond any health professional's primary education. Indeed, cultivating such awareness reveals the subtle dynamics of rank, as expressed through the ability to recognise and engage spiritual skills such as compassion, humility, kindness and tolerance.[39]

A positive correlation between spirituality and employee attitudes in relation to commitment, satisfaction and job involvement has been recognised.[40] From an interprofessional team's perspective, spirituality is a force not only for motivation and meaning[41] but also for cultivating empathic discussions, as well as ethical and holistic actions.[42] Spirituality, regarded as an intelligence, reveals how everyday relationships and activities can provide a deeper connection to meaning in life, and how they provide new perspectives for problem-solving.[43] It suggests that spiritual intelligence not only *is* something, it *does* something in relation to the demands of daily life,[44] which adds depth to our human engagement in life.[45]

Occupational intelligence is closely connected to spiritual intelligence, in that the everyday actions of human beings are full of meaning, which can also reflect a spiritual purpose in all areas of lived experience, including work. The concept of occupational intelligence[46,47] reflects the multiple ways that each member of a team can express their unique ways of *doing* in terms of engaging meaningful actions that actualises their human potential.[48]

The critical point here is that *what we do in life and the way that we live through our attitudes and values* requires keen awareness and cultivation of our human potential. These qualities are highly important and they need greater recognition within the context of IPL and IPP. Within complex working environments interprofessional team members will benefit from creating opportunities that make meaningful connections to the work that they do and the people they serve, including the well-being, performance and relationships within teams.

VIGNETTE: APPLYING SPIRITUAL AND OCCUPATIONAL INTELLIGENCES IN COLLABORATIVE PRACTICE

A team manager within an interprofessional team serving a multi-cultural community was challenged by a recent review of the service. Feedback from a focus group identified levels of frustration concerning a lack of cultural competence when receiving treatment from the team's practitioners. One community member from the focus group said: 'The health professionals we meet are well intentioned, but they do not consider the importance of different cultural or religious perspectives'. The team manager reflected on the feedback and realised that the professionals working within the team were also not a homogenous cultural group. The manager decided to set up some training so that the team could explore issues of cultural and religious diversity, to help improve competencies in this area. At the next meeting the team agreed that this would be very helpful. One of the professionals recounted a powerful learning experience that happened for them while working with a person who had strong religious beliefs: 'I was seeing this person on a weekly basis and they were struggling with their illness and adjusting back into society. The client told me about their spiritual beliefs and how it helped to keep them going when life feels overwhelming. I did not do much really, but I valued their beliefs and said to the client that I understood how important their beliefs and practices are to them'. As the client gradually improved, the professional eventually discharged the client from their caseload. The client said: *'What has been most helpful to me is how you valued the things that are important to me.'* The professional recounted: 'I learnt so much from this client, I recognised that the way that I practice has to include culture and spirituality, especially about what gives meaning to people's lives and how this impacts upon their health and recovery.' The vignette reveals a level of spiritual intelligence in the way that the health professional was attentive to the client, conveying depth and sensitivity in the interaction. The health professional also enabled the team to reflect upon cultural interactions with clients and how this is important for cultivating effective IPL and IPP.

INTEGRATING RANK DYNAMICS INTELLIGENTLY WITHIN INTERPROFESSIONAL LEARNING AND INTERPROFESSIONAL PRACTICE

The literature presented in this chapter, along with the vignettes, gives some indication of the important interplay between rank dynamics and the effective uses of social, emotional, spiritual and occupational intelligences for teams to unlock their interprofessional potential. Rank is not only hierarchical in terms of vertical structures that are evident in many organisations. It also has a horizontal axis, where people's experiences, knowledge, skills, attitudes, behaviours and so forth reflect difference and diversity. Integrating rank within interprofessional teams requires the cultivation of awareness of the diverse ways that people's knowledge, skills and experiences can be used. The development of rank awareness requires members to develop emotional, social, spiritual and occupational intelligences to engage the sometimes hidden and/or subtle dimensions of *interprofessional potential* within teams.

RECOMMENDATIONS FOR CREATING AN ENVIRONMENT THAT ALLOWS FOR EFFECTIVE INTERPROFESSIONAL LEARNING AND INTERPROFESSIONAL PRACTICE

➤ Effective interprofessional team-working requires members, and in particular team leaders, to recognise the different experiences, knowledge, skills, attitudes and behaviours that each person in the team possesses.

➤ The evolution of a team's interprofessional potential requires intelligent appraisal of each member's unique qualities and how these can best be applied to enhance the well-being of each member and the overall performance of the team, which is the very essence of creating an environment that allows for effective IPL and IPP.

REFERENCES

1. Department of Health. *Working Together, Learning Together.* London: The Stationery Office; 2001.
2. Department of Health. *High Quality Care for All.* London: The Stationery Office; 2008.
3. Department of Health. *NHS 2010–2015: from good to great.* London: The Stationery Office; 2009.
4. Department of Health. *Health and Social Care Bill.* London: The Stationery Office; 2011.
5. General Medical Council (GMC). *Tomorrow's Doctors: outcome and standards for undergraduate medical education.* London: GMC; 2009.
6. Nursing and Midwifery Council. *The Code: standards of conduct, performance and ethics for nurses and midwives.* London: Nursing and Midwifery Council; 2008.
7. Reeves S, Lewin S, Espin S, *et al. Interprofessional Teamwork for Health and Social Care.* Chichester: UK: Wiley-Blackwell; 2010.

8. Mindell A. *Sitting in the Fire*. Portland, OR: Lao Tse Press; 1995.

9. Barr H, Koppel I, Reeves S, *et al*. *Effective Interprofessional Education: argument, assumption and evidence*. Oxford: Blackwell; 2005.

10. Hammick M, Freth D, Reeves S, *et al*. *A Best Evidence Systematic Review of Interprofessional Education*. Dundee: Best Evidence Medical Education; 2007.

11. Reeves S. Using the sociological imagination in the interprofessional field. *J Interprof Care*. 2011; **25**(5): 317–18.

12. Wright Mills C. *The Sociological Imagination*. Oxford: Oxford University Press; 1967.

13. Department of Health. *Breaking Through: building a diverse workforce*. London: Modernisation Agency, Leadership Centre; 2003.

14. Department of Health. *NHS Leadership Qualities Framework: a good practice guide*. London: Modernisation Agency, Leadership Centre; 2004.

15. Faugier J. *NNLP Update: national nursing leadership programme, newsletter*. London: Department of Health NHS Leadership Centre; 2000.

16. McEwan B, Seeman T. Protective and damaging effects of mediators of stress. *Ann N Y Acad Sci*. 1999; **896**: 30–47.

17. Oshry B. *Seeing Systems: unlocking the mysteries of organizational life*. San Francisco, CA: Berrett-Koehler Publishers; 1996.

18. Morin P. Rank and salutogenesis: a quantative and empirical study of self-rated health and perceived social status [unpublished doctoral thesis]. Cincinnati, OH: Union Institute and University; 2002.

19. Stevens A, Price J. *Evolutionary Psychiatry*. 2nd ed. London: Brunner-Routledge; 2000.

20. Mindell A. *Deep Democracy of Open Forums*. Charlottesville, VA: Hampton Roads Publishing; 2002.

21. Collins M. Rank: understanding the subtle dynamics of rank. *Health Serv J*. 2004; **114**(5918): 31.

22. Collins M. Taking a lead on stress: rank and relationship awareness in the NHS. *J Nurs Manag*. 2006; **14**(4): 310–17.

23. Handy C. *The Hungry Spirit*. London: Hutchinson; 1997.

24. Bourton C. *A Management System Exempt from Power: learning to manage with consideration from others*. Basingstoke: Palgrave MacMillan; 2006.

25. Gilbert M. A theoretical framework for the understanding of teams. In: Gold N, editor. *Teamwork: multi-disciplinary perspectives*. Basingstoke: Palgrave MacMillan; 2005. pp. 22–32.

26. Hinshelwood RD, Skogstad W. Reflections on health care cultures. In: Hinshelwood RD, Skogstad W, editors. *Observing Organisations: anxiety, defence and culture in healthcare*. Hove: Brunner-Routledge; 2000. pp. 155–70.

27. Andras P, Lazarus J. Cooperation, risk and the evolution of teamwork. In: Gold N, editor. *Teamwork: multi-disciplinary perspectives*. Basingstoke: Palgrave MacMillan; 2005. pp. 56–77.

28. Myatt DP, Wallace C. The evolution of teams. In: Gold N, editor. *Teamwork: multi-disciplinary perspectives*. Basingstoke: Palgrave MacMillan; 2005. pp. 78–101.

29. Poder P. Empowerment as interactions that generate self-confidence: an emotion-sociological analysis of organizational empowerment. In: Sieben B, Wettergren Å, editors. *Emotionalizing Organizations and Organizing Emotions.* Basingstoke: Palgrave MacMillan; 2010. pp. 106–25.

30. Bornheim N. Organizational conditions for positive emotions in the workplace: the example of professional elderly care. In: Sieben B, Wettergren Å, editors. *Emotionalizing Organizations and Organizing Emotions.* Basingstoke: Palgrave MacMillan; 2010. pp. 63–83.

31. Fineman S. Emotion in organizations: a critical turn. In: Sieben B, Wettergren Å, editors. *Emotionalizing Organizations and Organizing Emotions.* Basingstoke: Palgrave MacMillan; 2010. pp. 23–41.

32. Burrill CS, West MA. The psychology of effective teamworking. In: Gold N, editor. *Teamwork: multi-disciplinary perspectives.* Basingstoke: Palgrave MacMillan; 2005. pp. 136–60.

33. Goleman D. *Social Intelligence: the new science of human relationships.* London: Arrow Books; 2006.

34. Goleman D. *Emotional Intelligence: why it can matter more than IQ.* London: Bloomsbury; 1995.

35. Goleman D. *The New Leaders: transforming the art of leadership into the science of results.* London: Time Warner Paperbacks; 2002.

36. Goleman D. *Working with Emotional Intelligence.* London: Bloomsbury; 1998.

37. Weiss JW, Skelly MF, Haughey JC, *et al.* Calling, new careers and spirituality: a reflective practice perspective for organizational leaders. In: Pava ML, Primeaux P, editors. *Spiritual Intelligence at Work: meaning, metaphor, and morals.* Amsterdam: Elsevier; 2004. pp. 175–201.

38. Rosenthal S, Buchholz R. The spiritual corporation: a programme perspective. In: Pava ML, Primeaux P, editors. *Spiritual Intelligence at Work: meaning, metaphor, and morals.* Amsterdam: Elsevier; 2004. pp. 55–62.

39. Culliford L. Spiritual care and psychiatric treatment: an introduction. *Adv Psych Treat.* 2002; 8: 249–61.

40. Benefiel M. Methodological issues in the study of spirituality at work. In: Nandram SS, Borden ME, editors. *Spirituality and Business: exploring possibilities for a new management paradigm.* Heidelberg: Springer; 2000. pp. 33–44.

41. Zohar D, Marshall I. *Spiritual Capital: wealth we can live by.* London: Bloomsbury; 2004.

42. Zsolnai L. Ethics needs spirituality. In: Nandram SS, Borden ME, editors. *Spirituality and Business: exploring possibilities for a new management paradigm.* Heidelberg: Springer; 2010. pp. 87–90.

43. Emmons R. Spirituality and intelligence: problems and prospects. *Int J Psychol Relig.* 2000; 10(1): 57–64.

44. Emmons R. Is spirituality an intelligence? Motivation, cognition, and the psychology of ultimate concern. *Int J Psychol Relig.* 2000; 10(1): 3–26.

45. Grof S. *Psychology of the Future: lessons from modern consciousness research.* Albany, NY: State University of New York; 2000.

46. Collins M. Engaging self-actualisation through occupational intelligence. *J Occup Sci.* 2007;14(2): 92–9.

47. Collins M. Engaging transcendent actualisation through occupational intelligence. *J Occup Sci.* 2010; 17(3): 177–86.

48. Collins M. Spiritual intelligence: evolving transpersonal potential toward ecological actualization for a sustainable future. *World Futures.* 2010; 66(5): 320–34.

CHAPTER 10

Changing demographics of the medical profession

Laura Bowater and Sandra Gibson

INTRODUCTION

The demographic of working doctors has changed since the inception of the National Health Service (NHS). Societal changes including the new social model of disability, the role of women and the advancement of a multicultural society have all played their part. This change is also reflected in the undergraduate medical student population that underpins the output of doctors into the NHS.[1] Recent legislation including the European Working Time Directive, the Equality Act 2010, and the new Health and Social Care Act 2012, as well as recent changes to the immigration policy are also affecting the demographic of the UK medical profession. Over recent years the number of medical specialties has also increased (65 according to the General Medical Council's (GMC) approved medical curricula) and the population of doctors practising within the United Kingdom has had to adapt to adequately fill these new specialties.[2] This chapter will describe how the demographic of doctors working within the United Kingdom has changed and adjusted in response to societal and legislative changes that have taken place in the United Kingdom since the establishment of the NHS.

DISABLED DOCTORS

Doctors living with a disability are in a unique position to empathise with and respond to the needs of the disabled community, as well as generating a diverse and inclusive workforce. Recent legislation is affecting disability within the working environment – in particular, the Disabilities Discrimination Act 1995[3] and the more recent Equality Act 2010.[4] It is estimated that in the United Kingdom there are more than 10 million people with disabilities and 6.5 million are of working age. Clearly people with a disability represent a large swathe of our modern society; however, this is not reflected in the number of students with a registered or declared disability applying for medical school or within the medical workforce.[5-7] In 2010–11, 6.2% of medical students had declared a disability, which is below the national average for students within higher education.[7] Accurate data on the number of medical practitioners with disabilities has been historically difficult to find. This was highlighted in the 2007 British Medical Association (BMA) report *Disability Equality in the Medical Profession*,[8] which discusses the issues that surround under-reporting and monitoring. For example, the NHS report *Quality Improvement Scotland* reported in 2011 that less than 2% of its workforce declared they had a disability.[9] The maximum value quoted in workforce monitoring for self-declared disability in an NHS trust was 3%, which is significantly less than the 17.7% observed in the local community.[10] Although some individual NHS trusts now report statistics, in line with the Equality Act 2010, it will take time for all trusts as well as the NHS to have reliable records.[4] It is hoped that the new rights and protection offered by the Equality Act will encourage clearer communication of disabilities between staff and employers and improve the problem of under-reporting.

The Disabilities Discrimination Act 1995[3] states that employers:
➤ must promote disability equality
➤ have a statutory duty to make reasonable adjustments within the workplace to support disabled doctors and medical students.

The inherent difficulty with the latter statement lies in the definition and interpretation of 'reasonable'. The GMC recommends that 'reasonable adjustments' should include adjustments to the physical environment, the selection criteria for posts and the conditions of service offered to employees. However, the BMA is quite clear that:
➤ 'reasonable adjustments' does not equate to a lowering of competency standards – rather, the *'methods of assessing or demonstrating these competencies can [...] be subject to reasonable adjustments'*
➤ if a doctor has a disability that could affect the health and safety

of themselves, colleagues or patients, the doctor should not rely on his or her own assessment of the risk that he or she poses. Instead, the doctor should consult a suitably qualified colleague and follow that colleague's advice about investigations, treatment and changes to individual practice to minimise any such risks as stated in the Health and Safety Act of 1994.[4,8]

Upon disclosure of a disability, a doctor is protected under the Equality Act 2010.[4] The current legislation within the Equality Act seeks to actively discourage discrimination and promotes equal opportunities for all doctors within an organisation. Despite this, it appears that the greater protection given to 'whistle-blowers' in the Public Interest Disclosure Act 1998 did not help address any under-reporting of disabilities or any associated discrimination. Despite this, disabled doctors continue to suffer discrimination and disadvantage that affects their career. This includes direct discrimination where reasonable adjustment to the physical environment fails to takes place. It also includes more indirect discrimination displayed through the attitudes, values and culture inherent in the workplace, including inflexible working practice, and unsympathetic or obstructive colleagues. In addition a widely held perception is that doctors should be fit and healthy; doctors who fail to mirror this norm face discrimination from colleagues and patients.[11] This perception contributes to a culture where doctors under-report disability within the healthcare environment. The result of this is that:

➤ even though the NHS is the largest employer within the United Kingdom, accurate monitoring of doctors with disabilities is not always taking place
➤ the number of doctors currently declaring a disability is an under-representation, making accurate estimations difficult
➤ this lack of accurate data is partly to blame for the reluctance of the NHS to build in adequate support and practices to meet the needs of disabled doctors.[8]

A different philosophical approach towards disabled doctors is developing. The medicalised concept of disability as a limitation to the activities of daily living is being replaced with the social model of disability that identifies that the limitations and barriers of the disabled are a manifestation of the exclusion and the negative attitudes of society towards the disabled (*see* Table 10.1).[12,13,14] Within this model there is recognition that disability can be ameliorated through

TABLE 10.1 Different definitions of disability

Source	Definition of disability
Medical model	Entails limitation in an activity of daily living[12]
Social model	An individual is disabled by society through attitudinal, environmental and organisational barriers and not as an inevitable result of his or her impairment or medical condition[8]
British Medical Association	'The end result of either mental, physical or sensory impairment or long term ill health which can limit functional ability'[8]
Equality Act 2010	A person has a disability if he or she has a physical or mental impairment and this impairment has a substantial and long-term adverse effect on his or her ability to perform normal day-to-day activities[4,13]
World Health Organization	'Disabilities' is an umbrella term covering impairments, activity limitations and participation restrictions
	An impairment is a problem in bodily function or structure
	An activity limitation is a difficulty encountered by an individual in executing a task or action
	A participation restriction is a problem experienced by an individual in involvement in life situations
	Thus, disability is a complex phenomenon, reflecting an interaction between features of a person's body and features of the society in which he or she lives[14]

changes in attitude at a societal, institutional and individual level. This adjustment is timely. The number of disabled doctors working within the NHS is set to increase as the age-specific disabilities associated with long-term chronic conditions such as type 2 diabetes, obesity and osteoarthritis also increases within the general population.[6,15] The GMC and the BMA recognise that good practice should be promoted within recruitment, training and work-based practice in order to support disabled doctors who work within the NHS and that this should be monitored. This should be driven forward through clear guidance, explicit organisational values and strong leadership.[8] The new Health and Social Care Bill has also led to the establishment of new organisations such as clinical commissioning groups and the NHS Commissioning Board that will be responsible for the design and the delivery of healthcare and services within England. The new bill clearly states that as these organisations are supplying services of a public nature, they must comply with the principles of equality outlined in the Equality Bill Act 2010.[16]

ETHNIC ORIGINS OF UK DOCTORS

Over the last half-century the ethnic origin of doctors working within the United Kingdom has undergone a significant change. There are two key reasons for this:

1. the steady immigration of doctors into the UK workforce to supplement the shortage of doctors in the NHS
2. an increasing number of home-grown, graduating medical students who are the children of first- and second-generation ethnic minority migrants.

Goldacre *et al.*[17] has tracked the ethnicity and the country of training of consultants working within the NHS from 1964 (the first year that the Department of Health maintained an annually updated database of UK consultants) until 2001. Their analysis of the data revealed that between 1964 and 1991:

➤ the majority of consultants (81%) were white and trained in the United Kingdom
➤ 3.3% of consultants had been trained in the United Kingdom but were non-white
➤ 6.2% of consultants had trained abroad, were white and had been recruited to work in the NHS
➤ 9.1% were non-white consultants who had trained abroad and had also been recruited to work within the NHS.

Between 1992 and 2001 this demographic changed, as the NHS continued to recruit doctors from Commonwealth countries (and beyond) to cover the shortfall of home-grown doctors. Vacancies were found in unpopular specialties such as geriatrics, psychiatry and genitourinary medicine and in challenging geographical locations such as inner-city primary care providers. Over this time period there was a 12.4% decrease in the number of white consultants who had trained in the United Kingdom, a 3.9% increase in the number of non-white consultants who had trained in the United Kingdom, a 3.8% increase in the number of white consultants who had trained abroad and a 5% increase in the number of non-white consultants who had trained abroad.[17] The number of non-white consultants training in the United Kingdom has continued to grow in parallel with increasing numbers of non-white graduates from UK medical schools (*see* Figures 10.1 and 10.2).[17,18] These data illustrate the pivotal role that migrant doctors have played in the development of the NHS. Many international doctors recruited during this time came to the United Kingdom intending to develop their skills and further their career before they returned home. However, the good career prospects, the value placed on their contributions to the NHS and the British public, and long-term shortages within the medical profession resulted in a net influx of doctors who have settled within the United Kingdom, raising children and buying houses.[17]

However, the role of internationally trained doctors within the United Kingdom is changing. This is as a direct result of a decision taken in 1997 by the British government to expand the number of medical school places offered in the United Kingdom to tackle the shortage of doctors within the NHS. There was also a growing awareness of the lack of ethical accountability associated with recruiting doctors from developing and third world countries, where there are fewer doctors per head of population, limited access to healthcare and a lower life expectancy. The changes to the Highly Skilled Migrant Programme in 2006 that allowed the immigration of highly skilled workers into the United Kingdom to seek employment opportunities has also made it increasingly difficult for doctors outside the European Union (EU) to find employment within the United Kingdom.[18] The introduction of new immigration rules in 2012, designed to tighten up the immigration policies towards migrant workers entering the United Kingdom, is likely to lead to a further reduction of migrant doctors from outside the EU working within the NHS.[19] In contrast, there is now a greater freedom for doctors trained within the EU to work within the United Kingdom. The reclassification of the tier system, the points-based system that regulates immigration into the United Kingdom, places a significant barrier to junior doctors from outside the EU progressing within the NHS.[20] These recent changes implemented by the UK government are designed to remove the post-study route into employment previously used by international students (including medical students) at a time when unemployment levels in UK graduates are increasing. The intention is to cap the time that migrant workers can stay in the United Kingdom at 6 years.[20,21]

There are still programmes designed to allow overseas doctors the opportunity to train in the United Kingdom for up to 2 years before using their experience to improve the health service in their home countries. These include the Medical Training Initiative backed by the Medical Royal Colleges, the English postgraduate deaneries, the NHS and the Department of Health as well as the International Sponsorship Scheme facilitated by the Royal College of Physicians in London.[21] However, the full impact of these new immigration policies on the medical workforce has yet to be seen. Currently, international medical students studying at UK medical schools have been built into the future workforce planning numbers of the NHS. Under this new immigration policy, these students will no longer be eligible to stay in the United Kingdom for longer than 6 years.

A quick perusal of the government-approved Shortage Occupation List indicates there are still medical specialties including genitourinary medicine, psychiatry and geriatric medicine that are continuing to struggle to attract doctors trained within the United Kingdom or the EU, therefore adding to the concern that the recent changes in immigration policy can potentially result in the NHS facing a shortage of doctors.[20]

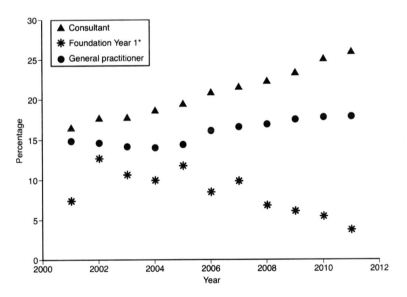

FIGURE 10.1 Change in the percentage of doctors, at three medical grades, who have qualified overseas (outside the European Union) between 2001 and 2011 (*Foundation Year 1, includes those classed as junior house officer)

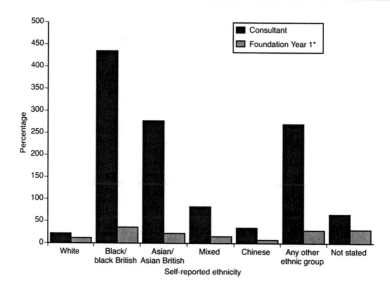

FIGURE 10.2 Change in the percentage of the self-reported ethnicity of doctors, at three medical grades, between 2001 and 2012 (*Foundation Year 1, includes those classed as junior house officer)

FEMINISATION OF THE WORKFORCE

Feminisation of the medical workforce is a reality. At the time of the inception of the NHS, medicine was a male-dominated profession and this was reflected in the make-up of medical students.[1] Since then there has been a gradual but steady reversal in the male-to-female ratio. By the late 1990s women were the majority of successful applicants to medical schools within the United Kingdom and by 2007 within the NHS:

➤ Forty per cent of the medical workforce were female.
➤ Forty-three per cent of female doctors were less than 35 years old.
➤ Specific specialties that offer career prospects compatible with maintaining a healthy work and family life balance attract a female workforce – these include general practice, paediatrics, psychiatry and public health.
➤ Fourteen per cent of consultants had part-time contracts and the majority of these part-time consultants (60%) were female.
➤ Twenty-eight per cent of consultants working in hospital and community health settings were female.

➤ Only 12% of clinical professors and 36% of clinical lecturers employed in UK medical schools were female.[22]

An increase in female medical students will lead to an increase of females in postgraduate training positions and ultimately an increase in female consultants.[23] Although the number of female staff reaching registrar level has increased over the past 5 years, this is not yet reflected in the rate of increase in female consultants (*see* Figure 10.3). Based on the number of female specialist trainees in 2007 and F1 trainees in 2002, we should be seeing current numbers of female consultants nearing or exceeding 50%.[24]

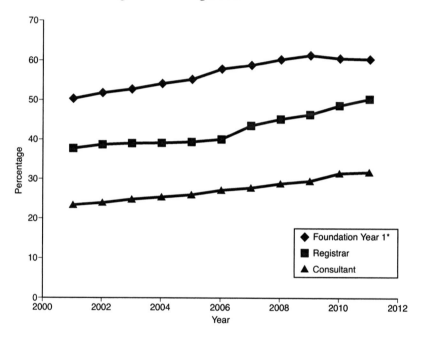

FIGURE 10.3 Change in the percentage of female staff numbers, at three grades, between 2001 and 2011 (*Foundation Year 1, includes those classed as junior house officer)

Although data suggest there are good retention rates among both female and male doctors, it is apparent that this gender balance shift brings associated issues that need to be considered within the workplace. Professional women are delaying starting a family until they have established their career. Currently, 43% of female doctors are less than 35 years old and may not have started a family. As more and more female doctors enter the profession, the percentage of doctors who may take a career break or seek part-time work in order to raise a family is set to increase.[23] The implications of this feminisation has been referred to as a 'time bomb'.[25] The concern is that those specialties that particularly attract females are facing a numbers crisis, as their female workforce are more likely to:

➤ take career breaks to start/raise a family
➤ choose to work part-time
➤ take early retirement
➤ choose not to work out of hours.

This projected decrease in the number of doctors on a full-time contract is arising in parallel with the recent implementation of the European Working Time Directive that requires doctors to reduce their working hours to a 48-hour week. This has necessitated employers finding solutions to a potential shortfall of doctors. These include designing more flexible shift work patterns or employing 1.4 female consultants for every one full-time equivalent post in specialties that attract a high percentage of female doctors in order to compensate for part-time working among female doctors.[23]

Women working in general practice are also filling the new position of the salaried doctor, created from the emergence of the new general practitioner contract, which facilitates part-time working. In 2005, 71% of salaried doctors were female, and of these salaried doctors, 64% were working part-time. This move towards salaried doctor positions is likely to have knock-on effects for women taking more senior or leadership roles in primary care. Women tend to become partner practice owners as they achieve seniority within the workplace, but the salaried doctor route makes this advancement much more unlikely which has implications for the future leadership roles of female general practitioners.[23]

Turning our attention to the hospital environment, leadership is evidenced by the role of consultant. A recent two-dimensional model based both on being more or less people oriented and on the ability to plan workload within the job has been used to map medical specialties, as shown in Figure 10.4. The percentage of women consultants tends to be highest in the specialties on the left-hand side of the figure that are more people oriented and with more 'plannable' working patterns (*see* Figure 10.4). It is clear that there are some specialties that attract a high number of female applicants and consequently have a higher number of female consultants, such as public health, paediatrics, pathology and psychiatry. If the general medicine specialty is examined in more detail, female consultants are much more prevalent in geriatric medicine and gerontology. Overall the surgical specialties recruit fewer female than male surgeons (fewer than one in ten) and only three specialised fields have a workforce with more than 10% female surgeons: paediatric surgery, plastic surgery and oral and maxillo facial surgery. The trend is for the younger female surgeons to attain consultancy rather than the older female surgeons who have been working for longer within the NHS (*see* Figure 10.5).[23]

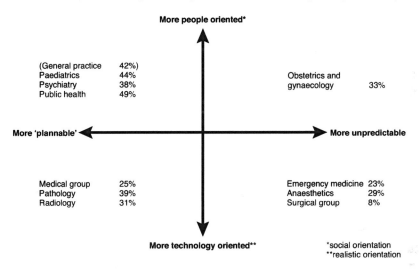

FIGURE 10.4 Specialty characteristics: percentage of female consultants and general practitioners, National Health Service England, 2007

There are areas where female leaders are still under-represented, and academic medicine is a prime example of this. This gender imbalance is also evidenced when female authorship on academic publications is examined. Although there is an overall increase in the percentage of female senior authors, it still lags behind their male counterparts, implying that there are gender-specific issues adversely affecting female authorship that may include family or caring responsibilities and discrimination within the workplace.[23,25]

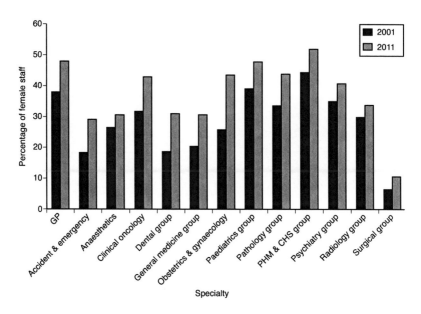

FIGURE 10.5 Percentage of female staff numbers in various medical specialties, in 2001 and 2011

In addition there may well be inherent bias in the top echelons
of the medical professions that increase the likelihood of failure
(or success) of those females who apply to senior positions within
specialties. Differences in success rates has been observed in the
application to, and pass rates for, a number of specialist training and
college membership assessments.[26,27] For example, the Royal College
of Physicians highlighted a need for further research within their
own postgraduate assessment systems to investigate both ethnic and
gender disparities.[28] This was evident yet again in the 2011 results of
the Royal College of Physician exams: UK female graduates achieved
the same pass rates as their male colleagues in only one of the four
examination results reported. Interestingly international female
graduates did better than their male counterparts.

SUMMARY

The NHS is constantly trying to balance providing a public service
with the provision of adequate training for new doctors. Historically,

balancing these requirements has caused difficulty when developing a workforce to fulfil both needs. The net result has been an underestimation of the numbers of doctors that need to be supplied through medical graduates. In the past this shortfall has been addressed by seeking doctors from abroad. This is no longer an easy fix with the new immigration laws and the challenges associated with estimating the number of EU doctors attracted to both UK training and consultant posts. Estimating and planning the medical workforce must also work around the uncertainties surrounding:

➤ the female workforce, including requests for part-time or flexible working and career breaks
➤ the increase of doctors with disabilities graduating into the workforce, and doctors who may now disclose previously undeclared disabilities that require workplace adjustments.

Finally, the new graduate medical workforce that is entering the NHS is also changing and may be housing its own difficulties when it comes to planning the future medical workforce. This includes an increase in the number of female doctors that may not necessarily translate into full-time working equivalents. Currently, it also includes international medical students who may not be able to work within the NHS upon graduation, leading to a shortfall in the predicted number of graduates moving into postgraduate training positions. However, the never-ending challenges of NHS workforce planning has the potential to generate future exciting and innovative solutions.

RECOMMENDATIONS

➤ Set aside protected time to allow individuals to complete trust and NHS workforce monitoring surveys and questionnaires.
➤ Foster a supporting working environment that encourages the disclosure of difficulties and open discourse on issues faced by the disabled in the workplace.
➤ When considering interviews, promotions, appraisal panels and those designing and carrying out assessments, ensure that they are as representative of the range of candidates as possible.
➤ Include diversity and equality champions within the organisations at levels where they are easily accessible to staff.
➤ Make sure that literature about the range of, and routes to seek, support are included in induction and within normal

communication channels rather than only becoming evident when problems or issues arise.

➤ Include equality and diversity as a rolling agenda item for departmental and organisational meetings.

➤ Include equality and diversity representative/s on organisational level committees.

➤ Develop a staff equality group.

REFERENCES

1. Gibson S, Bowater L. The shifting landscape: how undergraduate students have changed. In: Cavenagh P, Leinster SJ, Miles S, editors. *The Changing Face of Medical Education.* Oxford: Radcliffe Publishing; 2011. pp. 51–63.

2. General Medical Council (GMC). *Definitive List of Approved Single Specialities and Approved Subspecialities.* London: GMC; 2011. Available at: www.gmc-uk.org/Definitive_list_of_approved_specialties_and_subspecialties.pdf_45167060.pdf (accessed 3 July 2012).

3. Disability Discrimination Act 1995. Available at: www.legislation.gov.uk/ukpga/1995/50/contents (accessed 3 July 2012).

4. Equality Act 2010. Available at: www.legislation.gov.uk/ukpga/2010/15/contents/enacted (accessed 3 July 2012).

5. Health and Safety Executive. *Workforce Facts on Disability.* Available at: www.hse.gov.uk/disability/facts.htm (accessed 5 July 2012).

6. DeLisa JA, Thomas P. Physicians with disabilities and the physician workforce: a need to reassess our policies. *Am J Phys Med Rehabil.* 2005; 84(1): 5–11.

7. www.hesa.ac.uk

8. British Medical Association (BMA). *Disability Equality in the Medical Profession.* London: BMA; 2007. Available at: http://bma.org.uk/developing-your-career/becoming-a-doctor/disability-in-the-medical-profession (accessed 5 July 2012).

9. *Workforce and Equality Monitoring Report 2009–2010.* Edinburgh: NHS Quality Improvement Scotland; 2011.

10. Clark S. *Workforce Monitoring Report October 2011.* Manchester: Stockport NHS Foundation Trust; 2011.

11. British Medical Association (BMA). *Career Barriers in Medicine: doctors' experiences.* London: BMA; 2004.

12. Longmore M, Wilkinson I, Torok E, editors. *Oxford Handbook of Clinical Medicine.* 5th ed. Oxford: Oxford University Press; 2001.

13. British Government. *Definition of Disability under the Equality Act 2010.* London: British Government. Available at: www.gov.uk/definition-of-disability-under-equality-act-2010 (accessed 30 January 2013).

14. World Health Organization (WHO). *Health Topics: disabilities.* Geneva: WHO; 2012. Available at: www.who.int/topics/disabilities/en (accessed 3 July 2012).

15. Boult C, Altman M, Gilbertson D, *et al.* Decreasing disability in the 21st

century: the future effects of controlling six fatal and nonfatal conditions. *Am J Public Health*. 1996; **86**(10): 1388–93.

16. Department of Health. *Health and Social Care Bill 2011: equality analyses.* London: Department of Health; 2011. Available at: www.dh.gov.uk/prod_consum_dh/groups/dh_digitalassets/documents/digitalasset/dh_129978.pdf (accessed 19 February 2013).

17. Goldacre MJ, Davidson JM, Lambert TW. Country of training and ethnic origin of UK doctors: database and survey studies. *BMJ*. 2004; **329**(7466): 583–4.

18. Foster M, Rawaf S, Pelly M, *et al.* The UK medical workforce: sleepwalking into isolation? *Lancet*. 2008; **371**(9631): 2172.

19. NHS Employers. *Immigration Rules.* Leeds: NHS Employers; 2012. Available at: www.nhsemployers.org/RecruitmentAndRetention/International Recruitment/current-immigration-rules/Pages/IR-CurrentImmigrationRules GeneralIntro.aspx (accessed 3 July 2012).

20. Home Office. *Statement of Changes in Immigration Rules – WMS.* London: Home Office; 2012. Available at: www.homeoffice.gov.uk/publications/about-us/parliamentary-business/written-ministerial-statement/immigration-rules-wms (accessed 3 July 2012).

21. Skills for Health – Workforce Projects Team. *Medical Training Initiative (MTI) Guide.* Manchester: Skills for Health – Workforce Projects Team; 2009.

22. Elston MA. *Women and Medicine: the future.* London: Royal College of Physicians; 2009.

23. Dacre J. *Have we created an era of over feminism? Medicine: sexist or over feminised meeting* [lecture]. Royal Society of Medicine, 2011. Quoted in Khan M. Medicine: a woman's world? *BMJ*. 2012. Available at: http://careers.bmj.com/careers/advice/view-article.html?id=20006082 (accessed 3 July 2012).

24. McKinstry B. Are there too many female medical graduates? Yes. *BMJ*. 2008; **336**(7647): 748.

25. Sidhu R, Rajashekhar P, Lavin VL, *et al.* The gender imbalance in academic medicine: a study of female authorship in the United Kingdom. *J R Soc Med*. 2009; **102**(8): 337–42.

26. Tryer SP, Leung WC, Salls J, *et al.* The relationship between medical school training, age, gender and success in the MRCPsych examinations. *Psychiatrist*. 2002; **26**: 257–63.

27. Rushd S, Landau AB, Khan JA, *et al.* An analysis of the performance of UK medical graduates in the MRCOG Part 1 and Part 2 written examinations. *Postgrad Med J*. 2012; **88**(1039): 249–54.

28. *Membership of the Royal College of Physicians of the United Kingdom: annual review 2011–12.* London: Royal College of Physicians; 2012.

CHAPTER 11

Doctors as educators

Veena Rodrigues

INTRODUCTION

The education and training of medical students and medical and non-medical healthcare professionals on the team is a professional obligation of all doctors.[1] It is recognised that teachers have a powerful influence as educators and role models on medical students and postgraduate trainees. However, teaching skills are not inborn and consequently they need to be developed and nurtured by individuals in roles with defined teaching responsibilities. In order to facilitate teaching and learning, universities have a responsibility to provide staff development programmes to develop the teaching skills of new university appointees. For universities with medical schools, there is an additional requirement to provide staff development programmes for doctors employed within the National Health Service (NHS) who have teaching roles within the medical schools.[1]

Although there are many similarities between teaching in higher education institutes and medical education in general, the most important difference is that the patient lies at the heart of medical education, with good medical education ultimately benefiting patients. Recognising this, the Academy of Medical Educators has developed a set of professional standards for medical educators in the United Kingdom.[2] This framework includes a set of core values expected of all medical educators: professional integrity, educational scholarship, equality of opportunity and diversity, and respect for the public, patients, learners and colleagues. It also specifies the expected standards for medical educator competence in relation to knowledge, skills and behaviour at each level of their career. These standards define and inform the professional recognition scheme for medical educators in the United Kingdom and cover five domains: (1) design and planning of learning activities, (2) teaching and supporting learners, (3) assessment and feedback to learners, (4) educational research and evidence-based practice, and (5) educational management and leadership. It is expected that in future, achievement in medical education will be formally linked to the revalidation process for doctors being developed by the General Medical Council (GMC).[3]

THE CHANGING ROLE OF MEDICAL EDUCATORS: CHALLENGES AND OPPORTUNITIES

Over the past 2 decades there have been several advances made in the field of medical education. These include a move away from face-to-face teaching in the classroom to e-learning and distance learning because of technological advances; changes in the methods of delivery – for example, use of problem-based learning, interprofessional learning, and an increased emphasis on self-directed learning; and a change in the focus of education, moving away from teacher-centred teaching and learning and towards student-centred teaching and learning. This has resulted in a change in the traditional role of the teacher, which has now diversified into several areas of activity reflecting the complexity of medical education.[4]

Challenges facing institutions involved in medical education today[4-7] include:

➤ higher value placed on research over teaching at universities
➤ economic constraints pressurising clinicians to prioritise service delivery over teaching and requiring doctors to work in posts with little educational benefit
➤ changes to the clinical teaching environment and mix of cases in teaching hospitals
➤ variation in teaching and assessment across institutions
➤ poor profile of teaching compared with the other responsibilities of doctors
➤ lack of recognition for good teachers in terms of career progression
➤ lack of investment in funding for undergraduate and postgraduate medical education.

There is also anecdotal evidence of funding provided for medical education being used to employ researchers or conduct research. While the number of medical students in the United Kingdom has increased significantly over the past decade, the number of clinical academics, particularly in the clinical lecturer grade, has been declining with concerning trends in some specialties.[8] This has required many clinicians to increase their teaching responsibilities at a time when the NHS is under constant pressure to meet clinical service delivery targets. Changes within the NHS, the changing expectations and attitudes of patients and society towards doctors, and rapid technological advances also have major implications for medical education. There is a constant need for clinicians to develop and update their clinical skills, and to teach these skills to junior doctors and medical students. In addition, training reforms and the introduction of the European Working Time Directive have led to a shortened length of specialist training, with the result that training must be more effective to achieve the intended outcomes.[9]

For individuals involved in medical education, the major challenges[6,10,11] are:

➤ lack of training in teaching skills, supervision, giving and receiving feedback, assessment
➤ lack of knowledge of educational theory, motivational skills, assessment of competence
➤ lack of time and lack of flexibility of time for teaching and teaching skills development
➤ inadequate funding and support
➤ lack of recognition and rewards
➤ competing demands on time of patient care, administration and research.

Attempts to address these challenges have led to the development of medical education departments in most UK medical schools, a rise in educational research and scholarship, and the development and consequent availability of a plethora of medical education courses and qualifications. In 2005, the Walport Report recommended a new career structure for medical academics after consideration of the challenges affecting careers in academic medicine.[7] This included recommendations for increased opportunities to explore educational theory and practice for undergraduate medical students, the development of academic training programmes in specialties showing a decline in academic activity, and a review of academic career progression criteria for clinical educationalists at universities. Redressing the imbalance between teaching and the other duties of clinicians requires the development of a structured pathway using a competence framework, systems put in place to support this, a change in doctors' attitudes to teaching, and protected time for teaching for clinicians with this responsibility. Within universities, funding streams need to be transparent and with an appropriate balance between the dual responsibilities of medical education and research, so that research is not subsidised at the expense of education.

Individual doctors also need to make a significant time commitment for teaching and other educational responsibilities. Junior doctors in training have to deliver clinical commitments but protected time for education is essential. At the consultant level, there is a need to formally recognise teaching and educational responsibilities, the time commitment for this, and need for continuing professional development within individual job plans, taking into account both university and NHS commitments for clinical academics. For the purpose of revalidation, in future, doctors will have to regularly demonstrate that they participate in continuing professional development that covers the seven areas recommended within the GMC guidance *Good Medical Practice*, one of which is teaching and training.[3] To this end, they will have to keep up to date with educational development, be willing to teach colleagues and develop their own teaching skills.

Excellence in teaching can be promoted in institutions by using measures aimed at individual teachers, and those aimed at enhancing the learning environment within the institution to improve the quality of teaching, use an evidence-based approach to teaching and clinical practice, and encouraging educational scholarship.[12] In trying to implement new competence frameworks and faculty development programmes at institutions, it is imperative that the existing identity model of the teachers and the teaching culture within the organisation is addressed sufficiently in order to achieve successful implementation.[13] Recent increases in tuition fees at universities in England will have a significant impact on teaching delivered at medical schools as students become more interested in 'value for money' of the teaching received.

CHARACTERISTICS OF A GOOD 'TEACHER'

Harden[4] describes a model encompassing the varied roles of the contemporary teacher that could be used by teachers, and educational managers to inform and develop personal and institutional educational activity. These roles are classroom/clinical teaching provider, facilitator and mentor, assessor, curriculum and course planner, resource developer and being a good role model. Although these roles are often interconnected and are sometimes delivered simultaneously, it would be unrealistic to expect even the best teachers to be equally proficient in all the roles, as each requires different skills and aptitude. In practice, most teachers will take on a number of roles, often varying with time, experience and seniority.

A good teacher is one who inspires, supports, facilitates and enhances student learning by focusing on what students do and how they learn rather than just imparting information to the student.[4,14,15] Good teachers are enthusiastic, effective communicators, and involve students actively in the learning process. They create a positive environment conducive to learning, and they are aware that effective teaching involves consideration of the learning needs and interests of the students and directing their teaching to meet those needs. Good planning and preparation is essential for sessions to flow smoothly within the available time and to achieve the intended outcomes. In addition, it is reported that good clinical teachers use their medical knowledge effectively, and are able to develop clinical skills and clinical reasoning in their students.[14] Becoming a good teacher is a continuous process of planning, experimenting, reflecting and evaluating effectiveness as a part of professional development.

An outcomes-based approach to develop excellence as a clinical teacher has been described by Hesketh *et al.*[16] It covers tasks that all teachers should be able to do well, such as teaching small or large groups, teaching in clinical settings, planning, managing and evaluating learning, developing and using resources, and assessing trainees; how teachers should approach these tasks – that is, with an understanding of educational principles, using appropriate attitudes, with understanding of ethical and legal issues, using good decision-making skills and using evidence-based methods; and the professionalism required of clinical teachers within the NHS and universities, which includes personal and professional development as a teacher.

More recently, a broader framework linked to physician competence and applied to all those involved in medical education has been proposed.[17] This consists of core competencies in the areas of medical knowledge, learner centredness, communication and interpersonal skills, professionalism and role modelling, practice-based reflection and systems-based practice; and specialised competences related to designing, delivering and evaluating educational programmes, educational scholarship, leadership and vision, and mentorship and development of learners and faculty. Although this framework can be used to facilitate targeted faculty development, quality control and resource prioritisation, it does not address how the competences might be acquired or assessed.

THE DOCTOR AS A CLINICAL TEACHER

A good clinical teacher should be able to facilitate continuity of clinical experiences to students and assist them in achieving the objectives of their placements, give constructive feedback to learners on individual performance when necessary, and provide support to enable the professional development of learners. Modelling appropriate behaviours and the ability to give and receive feedback constructively is imperative in helping learners develop their interpersonal and communication skills during placements.[5] Clinical teaching opportunities are not always predictable, and teachers and learners must be also prepared for opportunistic learning in the clinical environment.

Learning about teaching is an essential component of the undergraduate medical curriculum. Doctors as professionals are expected to reflect, learn and teach others so that patient care is of a high quality. Doctors are also expected to be committed to lifelong learning, and be effective mentors and teachers in the workplace.[18] Despite the challenges of introducing new elements to already full curricula, several medical schools have developed innovative methods for introducing this within the medical curriculum – for example, developing reflective portfolios, delivering teaching sessions and presentations, completing student selected components on educational theory and practice, and intercalating to undertake formal qualifications in medical education.

A new work-based assessment has been introduced recently for junior doctors undergoing Foundation training.[19,20] Assessors are required to observe and provide feedback to junior doctors on their teaching and/or presentation skills and to assess performance in relation to their stage of training, in terms of preparation and use of resources, clarity of teaching, time management, knowledge of the subject and interaction with the group.

Within the clinical setting, the need to create the right learning environment, the ability to assess a trainee's learning needs, the ability to assess and give feedback constructively, and continuing professional development of consultant teachers are key themes highlighted by doctors as important to improving the learning experience, irrespective of their age, gender, chosen specialty, stage of training and type of hospital.[21-23]

PROFESSIONAL DEVELOPMENT

Although teaching can be an extremely rewarding experience, most doctors enter the medical profession to develop as clinicians and provide clinical services and only a few are interested in becoming involved in medical education. Clinical teachers have a vital role in helping medical students build their theory–practice links from classroom teaching to the clinical environment, and they are considered to be experts in the clinical setting. Very little support has been provided in the past to help clinicians to develop and improve their skills in this complex role. This has resulted in poor-quality teaching based more on factual recall and passive transmission of information often pitched at the wrong level than on active involvement of learners and development of problem-solving skills.[11]

Most higher education institutes require new appointees with teaching responsibilities to undertake formal teaching qualifications (at least a postgraduate certificate) during their probation period. However, despite GMC guidance on the educational obligation of doctors,[1] there is no formal requirement for medical graduates, or doctors in training who supervise and teach junior doctors, to attain a teaching qualification. Most specialties organise training programmes that cover areas such as on-the-job teaching, assessment of trainees, educational supervision, dealing with trainees in difficulty and appraisal of trainees, but these are variable in content and quality and are often voluntary. Very few training programmes have a formal system for accreditation and reaccreditation of trainers. A new framework for professional development of postgraduate medical supervisors of doctors in training has been developed by the Academy of Medical Educators in response to concerns about inconsistencies in training of postgraduate medical supervisors across specialties and deaneries.[24] The GMC has recently published new arrangements for the recognition and approval of undergraduate and postgraduate medical trainers in order to develop a systematic approach to high-quality training, similar to that used in general practice.[25]

Being a good educator implies the need to continually develop, maintain and refresh teaching skills. A good teacher also keeps in touch with developments in the field of medical education, experiments with new methods, and reflects upon the experience and the results to improve practice.[13] Reflection is seen as an important part of the learning cycle for turning experience into learning. Both reflection-on-action and reflection-in-action are commonly used tools for educators to prepare, implement, evaluate and develop new strategies to improve their teaching skills.[9,26-28] Although reflection on successes is important for incremental quality improvement, failures can provide an emotional impetus to improve teaching.

A range of methods has been used to evaluate quality of teaching delivered at universities and medical schools. This includes questionnaires completed by learners and teachers and focuses on a variety of issues such as achievement of objectives, choice of teaching methods, quality of audiovisual aids and other resources, and involvement of learners. Peer observation of teaching has also been used successfully as a means of professional development for teachers. However, these methods are more suited to classroom teaching. Evaluation of teaching in the clinical setting,[29] which has hitherto focused largely on demonstrating clinical knowledge, also needs to incorporate evaluation of teaching and interpersonal skills.

There is a need to provide doctors opportunities for development as medical educators side by side with their development as clinicians and researchers. Clinicians wishing to take on some teaching activities might find basic teaching skills training sufficient. However, for those who wish to take on a formal role in teaching and training, it might be advisable to have an academic qualification. In addition, for those wishing to contribute to the evidence base by carrying out educational research, research skills training would be useful.[6,30]

While individual doctors have a professional responsibility to develop and maintain teaching skills reflecting their level of involvement in medical education, universities and healthcare institutions also have a role to play in encouraging, supporting and facilitating the professional development of doctors involved in medical education.

EDUCATIONAL RESEARCH RECOMMENDATIONS

➤ Given that all doctors have a professional obligation to teach, and that teaching and training roles will be considered as part of the revalidation process[3] for all doctors in future, what are the current attitudes of doctors towards teaching? What implications do these have for teacher education and development?

➤ Clinicians use a range of methods to develop teaching skills. What is the proportion of doctors in educational roles who are offered or who undertake teaching skills training? What is the most effective method to improve clinical teaching skills? What components would the framework for the development process have? What implications does this have for healthcare institutions?

➤ Role models and mentors in academic medicine play an important part in inspiring medical students and junior doctors.[31] What is the impact of role models on attitudes to teaching and development of individual teaching skills? Could development and support of role models and mentors in academic medicine help in the recruitment and retention of clinical academics?

➤ Characteristics of good medical educators comprise both cognitive and non-cognitive elements. Can non-cognitive teaching behaviours be taught and if so, how? Can the effectiveness of these methods be validated? Which characteristics of teachers facilitate the development of clinical reasoning in students?

➤ A positive environment is conducive to student learning.[13,14,32] What effect does the design of the teachers' learning environment and departmental teaching culture have on the professional development of teachers?

➤ Several published frameworks are available to define outcomes and competences for medical educators.[2,16,17] How can medical educator competence be acquired? How can this competence be assessed effectively?

PRACTICAL TIPS AND TRICKS FOR JUNIOR EDUCATORS

Every new teacher has a steep learning curve in getting to know the students, the curriculum and the institution and in understanding his or her role. Simple tips for improving teaching competence can be obtained from self-help guides. Attending workshops carried out by competent peers or experts can develop teaching skills. However, a theoretically grounded and detailed approach to development is required to empower teachers to change existing perceptions and develop a 'teacher' identity.[12,33]

General points

A good teacher should stimulate, challenge, interest, involve and encourage learners, and understand their learning needs. Be flexible and prioritise your tasks. Identify the students' and your own learning needs.

Preparation

It is important to know who your audience will be so that you can plan the session accordingly. Prepare well, rehearsing if possible to get the timing right. Know your lecture venue and equipment; arrive early to check equipment and setting.

Delivery

Assess prior knowledge of learners in advance or at the start so that you can pitch the session appropriately; use a suitable style for the learning needs identified. Try to link your session to a previous session or to a specific part of the curriculum so that learners can see where and how it fits in. Open by sparking attention using a prop, a rhetorical question, a challenging remark or a video. Keep an eye on the time and avoid overload.

Presentation skills and interaction

Maintain good rapport and eye contact with the audience; include all, not just front rows. Use vocal variation, facial expression, movements, and gestures to hold the learners' interest and prevent monotony. Use audiovisual aids appropriately; make sure slides are legible and use good colour contrasts. Allow students time and opportunity to ask questions and answer questions honestly – if you don't know the answer, say so. Try to stimulate discussion among the learners.

Evaluation

Remember the learning cycle and its relationship to your own learning and development as a teacher. Learn to give and receive constructive feedback from students and peers; use the feedback to refine practice.

REFERENCES

1. General Medical Council (GMC). *The Doctor as a Teacher*. London: GMC; 1999.
2. Academy of Medical Educators. *Professional Standards (2012)*. London: Academy of Medical Educators; 2011.
3. General Medical Council (GMC). *Revalidation*. Available at: www.gmc-uk.org/doctors/revalidation.asp (accessed 22 June 2012).
4. Harden RM, Crosby JR. AMEE Education Guide No 20: the good teacher is more than a lecturer – the twelve roles of the teacher. *Med Teach*. 2000; 22(4): 334–47.
5. Gordon J, Hazlett C, ten Cate O, *et al.* Strategic planning in medical educa-

tion: enhancing the learning environment for students in clinical settings. *Med Educ.* 2000; **34**(10): 841–50.

6. British Medical Association (BMA). *Doctors as Teachers.* London: BMA; 2006.

7. Modernising Medical Careers Academic Careers Subcommittee and the UK Clinical Research Collaboration. *Medically and Dentally Qualified Academic Staff: recommendations for training the researchers and educators of the future.* London: Modernising Medical Careers; 2005.

8. Medical Schools Council (MSC). *A Survey of Staffing Levels of Medical Clinical Academics in UK Medical Schools as at 31st July 2009.* London: MSC; 2010.

9. Department of Health. *The European Working Time Directive: UK notification of derogation for doctors in training.* Leeds: Department of Health; 2009.

10. Lake FR. Teaching on the run tips: doctors as teachers. *Med J Aust.* 2004; **180**(8): 415–16.

11. Spencer J. Learning and teaching in the clinical environment. In: Cantillon P, Hutchinson L, Wood D, editors. *ABC of Learning and Teaching in Medicine.* London: BMJ Group; 2003. pp. 25–8.

12. Ramani S. Twelve tips to promote excellence in medical teaching. *Med Teach.* 2006; **28**(1): 19–23.

13. Van Roermund TC, Tromp F, Scherpbier AJ, *et al.* Teachers' ideas versus experts' descriptions of 'the good teacher' in postgraduate medical education: implications for implementation; a qualitative study. *BMC Med Educ.* 2011; **11**: 42.

14. Sutkin G, Wagner E, Harris I, *et al.* What makes a good clinical teacher in medicine? A review of the literature. *Acad Med.* 2008; **83**(5): 452–66.

15. Pinsky LE, Monson D, Irby DM. How excellent teachers are made: reflecting on success to improve teaching. *Adv Health Sci Educ Theory Pract.* 1998; **3**(3): 207–15.

16. Hesketh E, Bagnall G, Buckley E, *et al.* A framework for developing excellence as a clinical educator. *Med Educ.* 2001; **35**(6): 555–64.

17. Srinivasan M, Li ST, Meyers FJ, *et al.* 'Teaching as a Competency': competencies for medical educators. *Acad Med.* 2011; **86**(10): 1211–20.

18. General Medical Council (GMC). *Tomorrow's Doctors.* London: GMC; 2009.

19. Foundation Programme. *e-Portfolio.* Available at: www.foundationprogramme. nhs.uk/pages/home/e-portfolio (accessed 15 June 2012).

20. Foundation Programme. *Developing the Clinical Teacher: guidance for assessors.* Cardiff: UK Foundation Programme Office; 2011.

21. Wall D, McAleer S. Teaching the consultant teachers: identifying the core content. *Med Educ.* 2000; **34**(2): 131–8.

22. Rotem A, Godwin P, Du J. Learning in hospital settings. *Teach Learn Med.* 1995; **7**(4): 211–17.

23. Rolfe I, McPherson J. Formative assessment: how am I doing? *Lancet.* 1995; **385**(8953): 837–9.

24. Academy of Medical Educators. *A Framework for the Professional Development of Postgraduate Medical Supervisors.* London: Academy of Medical Educators; 2010.

25. General Medical Council (GMC). *Recognising and Approving Trainers: the implementation plan.* London: GMC; 2012.

26. Kolb D. *Experiential Learning: experience as the source of learning and development.* Upper Saddle River, NJ: Prentice Hall; 1984.

27. Kaufman DM. Applying educational theory in practice. In: Cantillon P, Hutchinson L, Wood D, editors. *ABC of Learning and Teaching in Medicine.* London: BMJ Group; 2003. pp. 1–4.

28. Schon D. *How Professionals Think in Action.* Aldershot: Ashgate Publishing; 1995.

29. Hays R. *Teaching and Learning in Clinical Settings.* Oxford: Radcliffe Publishing; 2006.

30. Hays R. Developing as a health professional educator: pathways and choices. *Clin Teach.* 2007; 4: 46–50.

31. British Medical Association (BMA). *Role Models in Academic Medicine.* London: BMA; 2005.

32. Hutchinson L. Educational environment. In: Cantillon P, Hutchinson L, Wood D, editors. *ABC of Learning and Teaching in Medicine.* London: BMJ Group; 2003. pp. 39–41.

33. McMillan W. 'Then you get a teacher': guidelines for excellence in teaching. *Med Teach.* 2007; 29(8): e209–18.

CHAPTER 12

Personal perspectives

Christopher H Hand, Amanda Howe,
Ian LP Beales and Ann Barrett

INTRODUCTION

In this chapter, four personal perspectives are presented, outlining how the changes discussed in previous chapters have affected the daily working, professional lives of two general practitioners (GPs) and two secondary care physicians.

PRIMARY CARE

Professor Christopher Hand qualified in 1971 and has been working as a GP since 1976, currently at Bungay, Suffolk. Until his recent retirement he was a Deputy Course Director of the Bachelor of Medicine and Bachelor of Surgery programme at the Norwich Medical School, University of East Anglia (UEA).

Professor Amanda Howe qualified as a GP in 1983 and has been working as a primary care practitioner since then. She is currently Professor of Primary Care at the Norwich Medical School, UEA; an academic GP at Bowthorpe Surgery, Norwich; and (at June 2012) Honorary Secretary of the Royal College of General Practitioners.

The changing face of general practice: a personal view of 35 years in Bungay, by Christopher H Hand

I qualified as a doctor in 1971 having trained at Clare College, Cambridge, and the Middlesex Hospital, London. After a 6-month senior house officer post at the Hammersmith Hospital I decided that hospital medicine was not for me. In August 1974 I became a

GP trainee in Ipswich – a decision I never regretted. I retired from general practice on my 65th birthday in November 2011.

The past

In October 1976 I joined a two-man practice in the market town of Bungay in Suffolk. My predecessor had been a GP in Bungay since 1933. The patients came mainly from Bungay, with the remainder coming from within a 5-mile radius of the surrounding countryside of Suffolk and Norfolk. The surgery consisted of five rooms, two of them for consultations. The patients arrived and waited their turn, which usually meant a wait of over an hour. Evening surgery often did not finish until 9 p.m. Country patients had their own surgery on market day and there was a surgery on Saturday afternoon. Only private patients had appointments. There was a lot of chronic visiting and 30–40 confinements a year both at home and in the local cottage hospital, All Hallows Hospital, which was owned by the local convent and had served the community for over 100 years. The hospital had an X-ray machine, which was shared with the local vets, and an operating theatre where minor operations, including tonsillectomies and adenoidectomies, were performed. There was also a maternity department and many of our older patients were born there. The on-call rota was tough: every other night and weekend. The GPs had 2 weeks' holiday a year and there was no locum cover. As my first partner said, 'The work was hard, but varied and interesting.'

In 1977 a new partner arrived, and the two practices in Bungay joined forces and converted one of the premises, The Beeches. The new surgery had 14 rooms including four consulting rooms and a treatment room. The team consisted of four full-time male partners, two practice nurses and seven employed staff. We had a health visitor, two district nurses and three midwives employed by Norfolk and Suffolk. Our list of patients was 9360, of whom 21% were over the age of 64.

Workload and premises

In a typical week during the 1970s and 1980s I would see around 175 patients: 140 in surgery and 35 on visits. I did two or three 2-hour surgeries a day with a 10-minute appointment system and had a single visiting session. I had a personal list and more than 90% of the patients I saw were registered with me. I had a half-day a week and worked 1 in 4 nights and weekends. I kept a detailed log of every patient seen from 1977 until 2001 and in that time I saw 138 942 patients; 95% were managed by me alone:

> 112 766 surgery consultations
> 26 176 home visits
> 6281 referrals to consultants
> 1466 admissions to hospital.

By 1985 the GPs were seeing about 450 patients a week and in 1987 we employed our first salaried GP to help us with patient demand. In 1988 the GPs were seeing 530 patients a week, and the practice nurses were seeing 150 patients per week (*see* Figure 12.1).

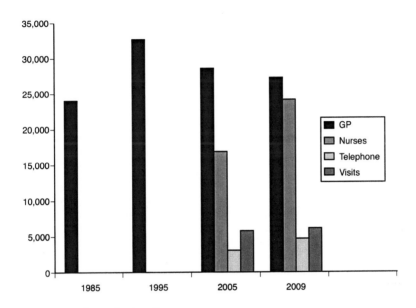

FIGURE 12.1 Consultation figures

After the New GP Contract in 1990, with all the extra work that it entailed, we soon ran out of space. We were seeing 630 patients a week. It was time to build a new surgery. One day a patient of mine said to me, 'Christopher, I want to buy the land for the new surgery'. As this was £100 000, I was amazed. She went on to donate £500 000 towards the project. The Bungay Medical Centre was completed in 2002 at a cost of £1.5 million. The building has 35 rooms on two floors and a lift. There are nine GP consulting rooms, five other rooms available for consultations, three nurse consulting rooms, an emergency room, an operating room and a phlebotomy room. There is also an attached pharmacy. The centre is run by a charitable trust, where most of the trustees are patients. Any profits are ploughed back into patient care, such as providing individual transport to hospital for patients having chemotherapy and radiotherapy.

The primary healthcare team has expanded exponentially since 1977 (Table 12.1) but the list size has only increased by 12% (10 641 in May 2012 with 25% aged 64 years and over). The increasing number of female GPs and the proportion of GPs working part-time reflect what is happening all over England. The nurses are rapidly catching up with the GPs in terms of the number of patients seen.

TABLE 12.1 The primary healthcare team, 2012

10 GPs (7 full-time equivalents: 7 female; 3 male)

GP registrar

Foundation Year 2 GP

10 Nurses:

        1 nurse practitioner

        5 practice nurses

        3 healthcare assistants

        1 community matron

5 District nurses

2 Health visitors

2 Midwives

2 Counsellors

Nursery nurse

Mental health link worker

Community pharmacist

Phlebotomist

Podiatrist

8 Receptionists

8 Dispensers

6 Secretaries

2 Clerks

Practice manager

Financial assistant

Practice development manager

Nursing administrator

Each week we offer, on average, 550 GP appointments and 450 nurse appointments, which is more than double what we offered 25 years ago. We do over 6000 home visits a year, just under half of which are to the 200 patients in the five residential homes and one nursing home that we look after. All these patients have complex medical needs and many have dementia. Twenty years ago most would have been cared for in hospital.

Although patients are registered with a GP, we no longer maintain a strict personal list system: continuity of care has declined. Approximately 50% of patients I saw were not 'my' patients, 10 years ago it was 20%; 20 years ago it was 10%. Continuity of record is not the same as continuity of person: most patients would prefer to see a GP whom they know and trust.

Local GPs found it increasingly difficult to cope with the increase in patient demand for out-of-hours care and this led to the development of our GP cooperative in 1994. One base was at All Hallows Hospital and we covered 35 000 patients. In 2003 we shared the night shifts with a paramedic based at Diss and the population increased to 70 000. In 2004 the base moved to Beccles Community Hospital and the population was 100 000. I stopped doing out-of-hours care in 2004, as did many GPs. Now there are two GPs on from midnight for a population of nearly 250 000. Just over 75% of the GPs doing out-of-hours work are male.

Computerisation and prescribing

Our first computer system, GP Base, was invaluable for repeat prescriptions, immunisations and screening. In 2000 we moved to EMIS. The disease templates have become increasingly complex and patients with multiple conditions are not well served by this system. The constant reminders of what I needed to do for the Quality Outcomes Framework were a distraction from the patient's agenda, and keeping my focus on the patient rather than the screen was extremely difficult.

The number of items prescribed has increased massively in the last 30 years, from 3000 items a month in 1980 to over 27 000 in 2010. Multiple drug regimens for coronary heart disease, hypertension, diabetes and asthma are partly to blame for this and are usually driven by National Institute for Health and Clinical Excellence guidelines. Advances in drug therapy during this time have been extraordinary: angiotensin-converting enzyme inhibitors, statins, proton pump inhibitors, long-acting beta agonists, selective serotonin reuptake inhibitors, and new generation antipsychotics come top of our prescribing league and were not available when I started in general practice.

Teaching and research

We started taking medical students from Cambridge and training GPs in the 1980s. I became a course organiser for the Norwich Vocational Training Scheme in 1982 and an associate adviser in 1992. The practice has taught all 5 years of students from the Norwich Medical School, has a GP registrar and a Foundation Year 2 doctor. The advantage of doing so much teaching is that most GPs are involved and it provides them with an important opportunity for professional development. The main disadvantage is access for patients.

We were one of the first practices to join the Medical Research Council General Practice Research Framework in 1978, for the mild hypertension trial, and we have been involved in over 20 studies. The research fostered an interest in academic medicine and so I started a Master of Science in General Practice at Guy's and St Thomas' in 1990. In 1994, I joined the School of Health and Social Work at the UEA to start a Master of Science in Health Sciences, and in 1999 I helped set up the new medical school where I was a deputy director until I retired.

Inevitably, being involved in teaching and research has meant I was less available to see my patients and continuity of care suffered. This is a choice that all academic GPs have to make and it is a difficult one. However, the personal and professional rewards have been enormous.

The future

The future of general practice is going to be strongly influenced by several factors, not least the current difficult financial climate, which is likely to continue for several years to come. The massive increase in numbers of staff, size of premises, numbers of appointments and prescriptions is neither sustainable nor affordable. Perhaps it's time to think radically about how we care for people, especially as the population gets older. Do we really need more drugs, more investigations and more referrals, or can we encourage the behaviours that really make a difference to people's health? No smoking, changing our eating habits, taking more exercise, and drinking less alcohol are preventive messages that are frequently not heeded, and yet we know they can make an enormous difference at low cost. GPs and nurses need enhanced skills to help patients change, but equally there needs to be financial as well as the health incentives for those who want to change.

Further political reforms are inevitable as every new government thinks they have the answer to managing the National Health Service (NHS). The Health and Social Care Act 2012 is just one step in the accelerating pace of change in the NHS over the past 35 years. The commissioning consortia will have to work closely with local authorities, not only because public health will be based there but also because health and social care are part of the same spectrum. This equally applies to the psychological services, which also need to be integrated.

With GPs now having a major role in the commissioning of care, it is clear that more patient care will take place in the community not only for convenience but also cost. Advances in technology may help this process. But who will be providing this care?

Practice nurses are taking over much of the work that GPs used to do, and with additional training could well do even more of their work. GPs, on the other hand, have retreated from some of their traditional roles, such as providing out-of-hours care for their own patients, and in the process have lost some of their professional status. This change, coupled with the loss of continuity of care makes the future of the personal GP uncertain. Other factors, including the difficulty in recruiting doctors into general practice and the increasing number of part-time GPs, may also contribute to a change in the future role of GPs. Those GPs who remain are likely to have more of a medical expert role in a primary healthcare team that will include other professionals such as social workers and mental health workers. Whether such changes will be as cost-effective as the old style of general practice remains to be seen.

A personal perspective by Amanda Howe

I have never felt particularly powerful as a doctor, which is odd, given the historical position of doctors being examined in this book, and my own career trajectory. I attribute my sense of relative powerlessness to four things. These are (1) my personal background, (2) my choice of professional discipline, (3) the human tendency not to perceive oneself as others do and (4) the learned professional knowledge that doctors are often powerless in the face of severe illness, individual limitations, and the unpredictable aspects of both biology and people.

Background: my parents were hard-working people who themselves had benefited from state education that altered their life chances, but it was definitely the aspirations of my own teachers that led me to move my career plan from important but less academic jobs to medicine. Me, a doctor? It took some time for this idea to become something I could commit to, especially because there was also the second doubting inner voice: 'You may be bright but you're a *girl!*' When I did get to medical school, less than 10% of students were female, and there was much sexist banter and explicit misogyny; but again, some redoubtable role models helped me believe I was both capable of becoming a member of, and indeed *needed*, in the medical profession.

History and culture, acting via education as this book shows, often lead to challenges to power and the status quo. Both the forlorn experience of shadowing busy doctors on ward rounds and my holiday work in a major cancer hospital (as a cleaner) sensitised me to the passiveness of patients and the complex hierarchies within and between different health professionals. Two trips abroad to Africa made me question whether the emphasis on hospital-based 'cure' was really the best way to help people be healthy, and the ravages of poverty and societal deprivation also made medicine look less powerful. The 1970s was a time of social change, but I could not analyse my experiences until I had the chance to undertake an intercalated degree, when modules in medical sociology, social psychology, and some specific case studies into mental health and women's health began to give me a conceptual framework to decide what kind of a doctor I thought was needed in society.

This, inevitably, led me to choose to become a GP – the lowest status medical discipline, without any compulsory postgraduate training requirement until the 1990s, and no required Royal College exit examination until 2007. This was, however, a discipline where one was in a less hierarchical relationship with patients and staff: close to the community, and able to lever on the causes of ill health. There were many other voices within as well as outside the profession looking for a different way to practise medicine; perhaps the best-known of my generation being David Widgery.[1] Being taught by Peter Huntingford and Wendy Savage[2] was also influential.

My experiences transferred into a conscious and happy choice to work in an inner-city practice in Sheffield, where we had some unconventional arrangements both for cross-practice collaborations to enhance services (an early type of federated practice[3]) and for our partnership arrangements. My salary was low by GP standards, but I had 6 months' paid maternity leave, which was almost unheard of for female partners, and I got paid for extra sessions worked as if I were a locum, which felt scrupulously fair! However, I (and my partners) were worried; we liked the GP training, but we were all really annoyed that at medical school we had had virtually no experience of general practice and the patients whose lives and health issues were so much a part of our daily work.[4] My future was altered by our collective commitment to get involved in as much teaching and training work as we could, and in due course to the opportunity to get involved with teaching on the university campus, where my enthusiasm and ability were rapidly seized on by the academic unit of general practice. A transforming moment was the interview to be a group tutor in general practice; a senior professor asked me if I had ever wanted to do research, to which I laughed and replied, *'No-one has ever asked me that since I said I wanted to be a GP!'* Within 6 months I was given access to research training as part of my university role, and I went on to do a doctorate, fulfil my dream of contributing to medical educational reform as a willing advocate of the General Medical Council's *Tomorrow's Doctors*,[5,6] and latterly became a member of the founding professoriate at a new medical school in the United Kingdom.[7,8] This medical school was part of a strongly multidisciplinary Faculty of Health Sciences, and both my clinical and academic practice have brought me to believe that doctors alone are, frankly, useless. This is because, however beloved and effective, one person cannot fulfil all the care needed by any patient over a lifetime; nor can one do really effective research single-handed.

This narrative hopefully has entertained and drawn memories and responses, but it may seem rather anecdotal, so let me make the key points explicit. Since 2009, I also have taken up a national role as an officer of the Royal College of GPs, which has given me close contact with the 'realpolitik' of health service reforms, and resurfaced a number of questions from my youth about the basis for, and the appropriate exertion of, power by doctors. Doctors' attitudes and roles may change because of technical and scientific advances; they may change because of the type and setting of educational input they receive; they may change because of the resources available to them, and how these are allocated. They will also be strongly influenced by the background from which they come,[9] the politics of their era, the role models available to them, the opportunity to innovate, and the values that drive them to undertake and sustain one of the most challenging professions. If these values are predominantly those of a highly rewarded and respected elite, whose craft basis is under their own control and which is dominated by commercial or technical priorities, then they will be a highly powerful profession. If the values are predominantly those of public service and a sense of moral altruism, albeit well rewarded for the effort, society will have a more reciprocal doctor who works in partnership with patients and other professionals. The impact of commercial imperatives and financial interests into healthcare alters the roles of doctors and their relationship with society. These are political, economic and professional choices. Any individual doctor or teacher will find these beyond their personal control – but our choices do matter.

SECONDARY CARE

Dr Ian Beales is Clinical Senior Lecturer and Honorary Consultant Gastroenterologist at the Norwich Medical School, UEA, and Norfolk and Norwich University Hospital. He qualified 22 years ago and has been a consultant for the past 12 years. He is also the Training Programme Director and Head of Specialty Training for the East of England Gastroenterology Training scheme and Deputy Director of the Norwich Endoscopy Training Centre.

Professor Ann Barrett is Emeritus Professor of Oncology at UEA and was formerly Deputy Dean of the Norwich Medical School, UEA, and lead clinician for oncology at the Norfolk and Norwich University Hospital NHS Trust.

The changing face of secondary care: a physician's perspective, by Ian LP Beales

I have worked for 11 years as an academic gastroenterologist in a large teaching hospital, but before that I spent 16 months as a consultant in a smallish district hospital. Superficially at least, the basic roles of a secondary care physician do not seem to have changed much over my career. The basic businesses of patient care, teaching, research, management and administration remain, although the actual delivery and organisation of these have developed in response to both medically driven and external factors, primarily but not exhaustively political and legislative.

Patient care

Even in my relatively short career, tremendous advances have been made in all areas of medicine. In gastroenterology we have new drugs, such as biologic agents for inflammatory bowel diseases and antivirals for viral hepatitis, which have significantly improved outcomes. We have more sophisticated imaging equipment. The technology of endoscopes and how we can use them has progressed to such an extent that it is now possible to treat and prevent cancers endoscopically, avoiding the need for such major surgical procedures as oesophageactomy. In parallel, our surgical and anaesthetic colleagues have developed minimally invasive surgery and perioperative management so that potentially curative surgery is now available to older and sicker patients.

The changes in organisation of care have been equally dramatic and possibly more difficult to personally deal with. During my training and early years as a consultant, I was used to having the traditional team or firm structure. A consultant had a registrar, a house physician (and a senior house officer, if lucky) who worked as one team on the same patients. The juniors often cross-covered other patients at night but everyone on the ward knew who was looking after Dr Beales' patients. Even without rose-tinted spectacles this situation had many advantages: continuity of care; longitudinal exposure to patients and diseases for the doctors in training, enabling them to learn about the evolution of disease and the response to treatments; the ability to build a relationship between consultant and trainees.

The various working time directive legislations have undoubtedly vastly altered the face of secondary care medicine. Although there are more doctors now, the traditional firm structure has disappeared. I now work in an emergency and inpatient gastroenterology team of eight consultants, four registrars, two core trainees and two Foundation trainees. All doctors except for the consultants work shifts; continuity of care apart from consultant input is non-existent. This means I certainly spend more time on direct patient care and have had to utilise the available teaching time with the trainees differently and more effectively.

Consultants today do spend more time directly involved with the immediate management of patients. When I trained, consultants consulted, they did a ward round once or twice a week but most of the day-to-day management was left to the registrars and senior house officers. One driver for this change was the move away from the firm structure, as outlined earlier, but mostly this was a laudable response to the perfectly sensible idea that patient care should be better if the most experienced doctors are making most the decisions and seeing the acutely ill patients as they are admitted. Now we have a consultant gastroenterologist on call 24 hours a day for advice or consultation and not infrequently emergency attendance at the hospital. There is much greater practical involvement by consultants in emergency admissions and it is not uncommon for me to spend all weekend, 8 a.m.–10 p.m., both Saturday and Sunday, in the hospital seeing patients or doing emergency procedures when I am on-call. We have seven consultants sharing our on-call rota, so the individual burden is not great; however, I can understand how it can be disruptive to family life, especially if one's spouse has similar commitments. It does seem to me that more doctors in training are now considering their career choice based much more on such factors than my cohort did; we tended to choose what we were most interested in. At present we have not got close to a full 24-hour service, there seems little doubt that working hours will extend in the future. We now run regular scheduled evening clinics to 9 p.m. and I am sure this trend will continue.

There has been an inexorable rise in specialisation. When I trained and qualified, we were in awe of the professor of medicine for his ability to see the big picture across all specialties and there is no doubt most of us as students wanted to aspire to that. This seems to have disappeared. Even when I started as a consultant I was 'physician with an interest in gastroenterology'; now we have not only passed through 'gastroenterologist with experience in general medicine' but have reached 'upper GI gastroenterologist', or 'pancreatic-biliary gastroenterologist'. Working as I do in a large teaching centre, my practice is almost entirely gastroenterology; we no longer do the traditional general medical unselected intake but have only specialty-based triage. I have mixed feelings about the march to such specialism so that now a patient can be referred to the 'wrong' gastroenterology outpatient clinic because that is the 'liver' clinic and not the 'oesophageal' clinic. I accept that for some patients, very specialist care improves outcomes but I remain unconvinced that this is necessary for everyone; especially those with co-morbidity, when taking an overall view rather than a single disease-centric view seems more appropriate. The drivers for this are not clear to me. Although a desire to improve patient care is a key outcome, it does seem as if specialisation is perhaps going too far and may partly be based in trainees and new consultants feeling less confident when working outside their immediate and slightly narrower comfort zone. Undoubtedly cross- and within-specialty referrals are increasing, but certainly, starting in the United States, there seems to be a bit of a backlash against this super specialisation, with the reinvention of the 'hospitalists' or what were called general physicians when I trained, as these seem to provide more holistic cost-effective care.

The demise of the firm structure has seen a rise in the wider team structure and a mushrooming of the number of specialist nurses. In my first consultant post we had two job-sharing stoma nurses in the department. Now I work alongside four nurse endoscopists, four stoma nurses, four bowel cancer screening practitioners, two nutrition nurses, two hepatology nurses, two inflammatory bowel nurses, two colorectal cancer nurses, three research nurses and separate nurses for oesophagogastric and pancreatic cancers. The management, organisation, mentorship and leadership of these sometimes disparate teams now forms a significant part of my own as well as many other consultants' workload.

Outpatient care remains the other mainstay of a consultant physician's workload and significant changes have occurred here as well, in both referrals and follow-ups. There are now multiple different routes whereby primary care can refer into our service: named-consultant referral, generic referral, open-access gastroscopy, direct access anaemia service as well as separate pathways for suspected oesophagogastric, pancreatic-biliary and colorectal cancers. The political initiatives and new resources surrounding improving cancer outcomes have had major effects of the design and provision of services. When I started as a consultant it was not uncommon to wait 6 months for a colonoscopy. Now a routine procedure waits only 4 weeks, and an urgent procedure waits 5 days. The downside of this has been an upsurge of protocol-driven medicine, which seems the only way to deal with the huge demand on the services. If a patient is referred with a suspected cancer, he or she will get the tests to diagnose or exclude that cancer, usually with a direct-to-test approach, and sometimes I feel that patients are not necessarily getting the explanations or assessment related to their symptoms they might otherwise want.

The outpatient workload and mix of cases have also altered since I first became a consultant. Some conditions have become much less common: antibiotics to cure *Helicobacter pylori* and potent antisecretory drugs have made uncomplicated peptic ulcer disease and peptic oesophageal strictures relative rarities, although acute gastrointestinal bleeding due to the more widespread use of anticoagulants and antiplatelet agents remains a major workload. The advent of highly active retroviral therapy has more or less abolished the previous major problem of diarrhoea in HIV-positive patients. In their place, other conditions have become much more common; these are a mixture of the diseases of affluence, alcohol and lifestyle (most obviously liver cirrhosis related to alcohol and obesity, as well as oesophageal adenocarcinoma), diseases that genuinely seem to be becoming more common, usually in some way related to immune system dysfunction, possibly related to the modern affluent world or the therapeutic drugs we use (such as eosinophilic oesophagitis or microscopic colitis), or iatrogenic diseases such as the rapid rise in radiation proctitis consequent on increased prostate cancer screening. Probably the biggest changes in outpatient workload have been the increased referrals of patients with problems related to ageing and degeneration and the otherwise 'worried well'. Problems related to ageing, co-morbidities and dementia such as constipation, faecal incontinence and diverticular disease are much more commonly seen now. Although the management of irritable bowel syndrome and other related conditions without objective organic pathology has always been a mainstay of gastroenterologists, I have noticed a vast increase in the number of referrals 'just in case', when previously mild symptoms and, indeed, national guidelines would not have usually instigated a referral. I am unsure whether this results from a decreased confidence in primary care to manage such patients, increased consumerism among patients or the result of providing a more rapid and accessible service that simply encourages more usage.

Administration and management

The various administration and management activities do seem to have grown in recent years. Last year I spent an average of 11.4 hours per week on the various tasks that would be encompassed within this, not immediately related to patient care. At the same time, there is considerably more management oversight over what consultants actually spent their time doing. Money, funding and expenditure are now much higher up the agenda and are usually the first things anyone mentions when discussing any new developments.

I have had to acquire and then refine the skills for negotiating through these difficult situations and, like many physicians, I have developed much better business sense, not only how to write a business plan and run a department like a business but also a much keener idea of how much my time is worth.

Since I have been a consultant, there has been an explosion in so-called clinical governance. This was mainly externally driven in response to primarily the Bristol-Heart, Shipman and Alder Hey events. In practice, I do not think these have had a great effect on me personally, apart from the time I spend generating paperwork. All good practitioners and units have been auditing their own practice and outcomes for as long as I can remember. We have become much more formalised in our approach to clinical and financial governance, and this I think is a positive development. Now for one afternoon per month, the whole gastroenterology department stops routine work and reviews audit, performance, plans and critical incidents. It is probably critical incident reporting that has caused the most culture change in recent years. The model often held up is the airline industry, and although I feel we have a way to go before we have free and transparent incident reporting and follow-up, progress is definitely being made. Most clinical incidents are a multifactorial combination of smaller factors and we have embraced examining and rectifying these in detail.

I would expect that revalidation will be the next biggest change to my administrative burden. As yet, no one really knows how this will work, but the processes do seem unnecessarily bureaucratic and unwieldy. Last year, just collecting the data and information required for my annual appraisal that will inform revalidation took about 100 hours, and my Royal College estimates that actually doing all the work for revalidation will actually require 6 hours per week, not including study leave. While I am sure that every patient deserves to know that their doctor is competent and has an appropriate licence to prescribe, the processes to provide these data are not yet in place as a viable system. I am sure these will be refined in time, but in the short and intermediate terms this does seem to have increased administration disproportionately.

Overall I have no doubt that the administrative burden associated with being a consultant physician has increased, even for those not in specific management roles. The breadth and number of tasks have increased, and in many situations these are not always in the skill set developed during undergraduate or postgraduate training and this has required development of these as a consultant.

The future

It seems almost impossible to even try to predict the future. After all, 10 years ago I would not have predicted we would have the national Bowel Cancer Screening Programme or the National Endoscopy Training Programme, both not only fully functional but also recognised throughout the world for their effectiveness. This shows what changes can be achieved with significant political will behind them. Clearly now in 2012 the NHS is at a crossroads, with the dissolution of Strategic Health Authorities and Primary Care Trusts and new practice-based commissioning on the horizon, as well as the spectre of 'any willing provider' in the market to supply healthcare services, there is a real danger that care will become even more fragmented and less holistic. The exact future and shape of hospital medicine and the work of consultant physicians is likely to evolve somewhat. Hospitals are expensive and complex organisations and consultants are flexible and highly qualified employees, although there seems significant move to narrower and narrower niches in expertise and work. I hope we see greater integration and organisation between primary and secondary care and more emphasis on quality and less purely on cost. It seems likely there will be a continued move towards more ambulatory care and care nearer to patients' homes, but common sense says that with the economies of scale and the technological support intrinsic to modern hospital medicine, it will not be viable to devolve that much to community settings. It seems inevitable that evening and weekend working will become the norm, but this will require more doctors and adequate funding.

Key points
➤ There have been major therapeutic advances and new, expensive drugs will continue to emerge.
➤ The organisation of the medical team has changed dramatically, but consultants have an essential role in leading these larger, multidisciplinary teams effectively.
➤ Consultant gastroenterologists (and probably most physicians) spend an increasing amount of time on emergency and unsocial hours work; this will have important ramifications for doctors' career choices in the future.
➤ Provision of outpatient services has changed dramatically. With more protocol-driven and straight-to-test referrals and significantly less chronic disease follow-up.
➤ Demands for training and teaching often conflict with service demands.
➤ Business planning and financial management are essential parts of a consultant's role; these skills need careful mentoring and development.

➤ We have seen an upsurge in activities related to clinical governance and the work required for revalidation seems as if it will take yet more time.

The changing role of the doctor and its impact on training and education of doctors: a secondary care perspective, by Ann Barrett

My experience of learning, practising, teaching and managing in medical practice spans half a century, over which time many fashions have come and gone. Government and professional initiatives have loaded my bookshelves with weighty reports, to some of which latterly I have been privileged to contribute. Working patterns have been adjusted to improve training and meet the requirements of our commitments to Europe. Doctors have lost and regained influence in managing healthcare organisation and resources. More effective treatments and increasing specialisation have had a huge impact on how doctors work.

My training began in the 1960s in one of the oldest medical schools of London – a monastic foundation, the ethos of which still seems to pervade the square and fountain around which, in my day, patients would be wheeled in their beds to provide variety for them in the long weeks of their hospital stay. How desperate were my pleas as a patient to be allowed home after 6 weeks of bed rest and traction in an orthopaedic ward, for a condition for which, 25 years later, I could be discharged on the first post-operative day.

I finished my career in one of the newest medical schools where, for a few glorious years before retirement (although subject to strict scrutiny by the General Medical Council (GMC) because it was a brand new medical school), we were able to experiment with new criteria for entry, new integrated ways of teaching and a patient case-based curriculum, which seemed to meet exactly the requirements of the career in which I had enjoyed working for so long.

Changes in selection processes over the years have reflected varying emphases on different qualifications for entry to medical school. First BM (undergraduate medical course), a course which taught physics, chemistry and biology to A-level standard in 1 year, used to give an opportunity for those who for some reason had not devoted themselves to the study of biology or whatever science was considered foundational. I had an entrance scholarship in Latin and Greek, which made learning all the new words much easier for me than others for whom the sense was not obvious. A notable member of our course, known affectionately as Grandpa, came from teaching and was able to help us direct our learning effectively. Forty years later, at the UEA, we rediscovered the gains that come from admitting students with a wide background of skills and experience.

The totally unstructured interview by which I gained my coveted place at medical school was replaced, when I was interviewing instead of being interviewed, by the skills stations; with little opportunity for the revealing individual questioning with which we used to think we could detect the person who would not make it. I still could not help looking for predictive value in some experience which was more personal – I thought that having worked in a care home might reflect some essential quality – though perhaps only for my sort of caring, empathetic doctor, not necessarily for a highly skilled technician or researcher.

The basis of my training was a knowledge-based approach, studying each subject individually. Learning by rote was principally accomplished independently and the large amount of time devoted to anatomy dissection is memorable only as a highly sociable activity with lots of laughter. Lectures on the core subjects of anatomy, biochemistry and physiology were the only points of contact with staff. Later, when we became clinical, time was spent erratically within 'the firm' to which we were assigned. Our learning was dependent on the interests of the consultant and whichever patients happened to be in the ward at that time. It seems incredible now that we had no exposure to general practice at all during our training. This is a marked difference in medical training from the UEA course in which GPs play a major role and students spend a day a week in practice from the start of the course.

Now that so much more is known about normal physiology and body functioning, it is impossible to retain by rote all the information that is known and relevant to each disease entity. Nor is it necessary to learn it since it is all accessible information on the internet. The biggest change was in the use of problem-based learning (PBL) to integrate all the relevant scientific and other knowledge needed to look after a particular patient – a much more practical approach, although for the purist (or Specialist Scientist!) there was a risk of lowering the standard of knowledge and not having a joined-up understanding.

For my generation, diagnosis was of paramount importance and we were taught that if we did not know the diagnosis by the end of history taking, we probably never would. Three-dimensional imaging and biomarker studies have changed that so that now it is guidelines and audit of returns from imaging studies that determine the process of arriving at a diagnosis. However, for the treatment of cancer (and other diseases of which I know less) the possibilities of accurate diagnosis and effective intervention have increased dramatically from these new technologies and it is as important to teach the principles of investigation as old-fashioned clinical diagnosis.

The firm system has given way paradoxically both to more individualistic working, because of new shift working patterns, and to greater team collaboration. Often a doctor on night duty will not see other members of the team apart from another peer at handover. The multidisciplinary team has formalised interaction between specialist disciplines of doctors and other healthcare workers. In breast cancer treatment it has been shown to improve some disease outcomes, or, at the least, the likelihood of the patient getting what is considered to be the right treatment. However, large numbers of healthcare professionals need to attend these meetings to meet targets that are not concerned primarily with improving patient experience or survival. The doctor–ward sister axis that ruled hospital practice has disappeared and continuity of care is a constant challenge. With a much larger number of people being involved in any decision about a patient, there is a problem in communicating and implementing decisions effectively and speedily. Often patients have to wait for news that they could previously have been told immediately.

This way of working also has a big impact on how we need to teach medical students. Interprofessional learning was part of the new curriculum at UEA in which PBL cases were discussed and worked on together by different healthcare professionals. These sessions were not popular initially. In spite of our best efforts, people seemed to come with built-in prejudices. Some were intimidated from contributing; others were irritated at the slowness of the process and tried to do it all themselves. It was hard to foster the mutually appreciative co-working that can be experienced when meeting during actual patient care, and status battles were not easily removed in spite of this approach. However, the negotiation skills needed for consensual decision-making were undoubtedly appropriately developed in PBL and interprofessional learning.

The management of health service resources seems to have become a much more high-profile and time-consuming business over the years. The half-century cycle of experimentation with one sort of medical director to another, one sort of funding to another does not seem to have solved all the problems. However, we all are probably now aware of the costs of things, competing pressures on resources, the need for rationing. Should we now be teaching all medical students elements of management or is it more appropriately an area of postgraduate training for those who show aptitude and interest? We are all required to manage resources and staff responsibly and to seek constantly for ways of improving the service and patient care. PBL made it possible to address these issues, although there was a tendency for fairly standardised approaches to management issues to be developed by some students and then applied to all cases being considered. We tried to teach the ethics of managing resource limitations, making realistic costings of service developments and the need for personal responsibility, as well as constantly encouraging students to keep looking for ways of improving things by individual effort, process redesign and bright ideas.

Work patterns have changed from those where continuity of service was the driver. We were on-call for all weekdays and alternate nights and weekends in a community where we lived and ate all our meals! We were even brought morning tea in bed by the residency staff. We had company as we worked, and we had support when things were difficult. We saw the outcome of our actions and learned about the natural history of disease. Because of pressures on beds, so many more available treatments and the number of people involved in decision-making, there is no time now to wait and see what will happen, which used to be a useful approach in those with chronic or terminal illness. Patients were in hospital for long periods of time and we got to know them and enjoy their confidences and the concerns of their lives. When the consultant asked, we knew the test results; we had ordered them and checked them. The ward nurse knew all the bits in between when we had not been there. Now it seems much harder and less satisfying for junior doctors. They are not there when the patient comes in and they will not be there when the patient goes home. Junior doctors may not get to teaching; if they are on the nightshift they may have to deal alone with things going wrong, just being summoned to account for their actions rather than being supported through the incident. Certainly, patients hardly ever know who is who, in spite of name badges and regular introductions. The growth of trust, which leads to patients sharing sensitive information, is more difficult. New skills of handover, inevitably passing on only summary points, have replaced in-depth personal relationships. Appointment of a key worker is the most recent attempt to restore the continuity whose loss the medical profession, and the patients, deplore.

Old hierarchies have disappeared and the role of most healthcare workers has changed substantially. Interprofessional working, now an essential skill and usually very rewarding, can be problematic where there is an overlap of roles. There are not usually difficulties between physiotherapist and doctor, or speech therapist and nurse, as the skills of the other are obvious and different, but the 'academisation' of nursing can make the nurse–doctor interface problematic if hierarchy and status remain too important in individual ways of thinking. Information giving to patients requires extra care when many different people are contributing. Changing demographics may have an influence too, as different cultural groups may have varying expectations of good practice. There are more non-white staff, female staff, secular staff and staff of other strong faith, than ever before, all with different life views that may impact on human rights issues and ethics. Some of the core assumptions of my practice were challenged when I had to teach groups of students in a module on human rights as part of their 'Studies outside medicine' course. The concept of the GMC Good Doctor was certainly more familiar to them than that of the Good Samaritan.

Teaching by doctors often conflicts with their responsibilities for patient care, research or management and pressures of time seem to increase relentlessly. Teaching by clinicians is important in spite of these pressures as they can use experience and personal example to press home teaching points. They act as role models and may have more credibility with students than other healthcare workers, particularly important in giving value to the teaching of 'soft subjects' such as communications skills and ethics.

Performance monitoring has become more formalised. I only once saw a member of staff individually for discussion of my progress during my whole undergraduate career, and that was when I failed an exam, but now there is a complex and appropriate network of support. What is still unresolved is how to deal with the student who seems to everyone to be unsuitable for medicine, whether or not academically capable. If they cross GMC boundaries or fail exams there is no problem, but lack of commitment, laziness, selfishness and lack of empathy are very difficult to deal with, although we sometimes know we are failing their future colleagues by not doing so. There is still a need for exit routes from medical training without any stigma.

Everything seems to be getting more difficult and demanding. We are more and more regulated. What delights me still is that enthusiastic, clever, interesting, kind doctors are being produced by our imperfect education systems and they are still taking initiatives to improve treatment and care of patients even though their working conditions, training and practice are subject to so much more regulation than we were used to.

REFERENCES

1. Widgery D. *Some Lives: a GP's East End.* London: Sinclair Stevenson; 1991.
2. Savage W. *Birth and Power: a savage enquiry revisited.* London: Middlesex University Press; 2007.
3. Royal College of General Practitioners (RCGP). *The Future Direction of General Practice: a roadmap.* London: RCGP; 2007. Available at: www.rcgp.org.uk/policy/rcgp-policy-areas/future-direction-of-general-practice-a-roadmap.aspx (accessed 6 February 2013).
4. Howe A. Patient-centred medicine through student-centred teaching: a student perspective on the key impacts of community-based learning in undergraduate medical education. *Med Educ.* 2001; **35**(7): 666–72.
5. General Medical Council (GMC). *Tomorrow's Doctors.* London: GMC; 1993.
6. Howe A, Campion P, Searle J, *et al.* New perspectives: approaches to medical education at four new UK medical schools. *BMJ.* 2004; **329**(7461): 327–31.
7. Howe A, Hand C. The challenge of doing things differently: one new medical school's vision of primary care education. *Educ Prim Care.* 2002; **13**(2): 205–321.
8. Howe A. Has a decade made a difference? The contribution of UK primary care to basic medical training in 2004. *Educ Prim Care.* 2005; **16**(1): 10–19.
9. Milburn A. *Unleashing Aspiration: the final report of the Panel on Fair Access to the Professions.* London: Cabinet Office; 2009.

Index

Entries in **bold** denote figures and tables.

CPD with Radcliffe

You can now use a selection of our books to achieve CPD (Continuing Professional Development) points through directed reading.

We provide a free online form and downloadable certificate for your appraisal portfolio. Look for the CPD logo and register with us at: www.radcliffehealth.com/cpd

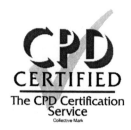

CERTIFIED
The CPD Certification
Service
Collective Mark